Atlas of
CONTRACEPTION

Atlas of
CONTRACEPTION
Second Edition

Edited by

Pramilla Senanayake MBBS PhD FRCOG FACOG FRSM FSLCOG
International Consultant in Sexual and Reproductive Health
Colombo
Sri Lanka

and

Malcolm Potts MB BChir PhD FRCOG
Bixby Professor of Population and Family Planning
School of Public Health
University of California
Berkeley, CA
USA

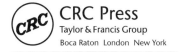

CRC Press is an imprint of the
Taylor & Francis Group, an **informa** business

CRC Press
Taylor & Francis Group
6000 Broken Sound Parkway NW, Suite 300
Boca Raton, FL 33487-2742

First issued in paperback 2019

© 2008 by Taylor & Francis Group, LLC
CRC Press is an imprint of Taylor & Francis Group, an Informa business

No claim to original U.S. Government works

ISBN-13: 978-1-84214-305-6 (hbk)
ISBN-13: 978-0-367-38748-8 (pbk)

This book contains information obtained from authentic and highly regarded sources. While all reasonable efforts have been made to publish reliable data and information, neither the author[s] nor the publisher can accept any legal responsibility or liability for any errors or omissions that may be made. The publishers wish to make clear that any views or opinions expressed in this book by individual editors, authors or contributors are personal to them and do not necessarily reflect the views/opinions of the publishers. The information or guidance contained in this book is intended for use by medical, scientific or health-care professionals and is provided strictly as a supplement to the medical or other professional's own judgement, their knowledge of the patient's medical history, relevant manufacturer's instructions and the appropriate best practice guidelines. Because of the rapid advances in medical science, any information or advice on dosages, procedures or diagnoses should be independently verified. The reader is strongly urged to consult the relevant national drug formulary and the drug companies' and device or material manufacturers' printed instructions, and their websites, before administering or utilizing any of the drugs, devices or materials mentioned in this book. This book does not indicate whether a particular treatment is appropriate or suitable for a particular individual. Ultimately it is the sole responsibility of the medical professional to make his or her own professional judgements, so as to advise and treat patients appropriately. The authors and publishers have also attempted to trace the copyright holders of all material reproduced in this publication and apologize to copyright holders if permission to publish in this form has not been obtained. If any copyright material has not been acknowledged please write and let us know so we may rectify in any future reprint.

A CIP record for this book is available from the British Library.

Library of Congress Cataloging-in-Publication Data available on application

**Visit the Taylor & Francis Web site at
http://www.taylorandfrancis.com**

**and the CRC Press Web site at
http://www.crcpress.com**

Contents

Preface   vii

Acknowledgment   viii

1   Introduction   1

2   Rationale for family planning   5

3   History of family planning   21

4   Human sexuality, including female reproduction and male physiology   27

5   Service delivery   33

6   Hormonal contraception   39

7   Condoms   57

8   Female barrier contraception and spermicides   61

9   Intrauterine devices   67

10 Periodic abstinence and coitus interruptus   71

11 Voluntary surgical contraception   77

12 Contraception for special groups   83

13 Abortion   95

14 AIDS   101

15 New methods   107

16 Conclusions   111

Index   115

Preface

Over the past two decades, family planning and reproductive health have become recognized as a medical specialty with professional organizations, peer-reviewed journals, and national and international meetings. It was not always so. There could not have been an atlas of this type in 1950, and even in 1980 it might have looked very different.

Family planning and reproductive health is a branch of preventive medicine that can have a profound impact on the health of women and their children. Like many other aspects of medicine, certain contraceptive choices require surgical or clinical skills in order to be used correctly. For some couples with chronic sickness or inheritable diseases, family planning advice is an intrinsic part of comprehensive patient care. Physicians have also taken a leadership role in family planning because they often see the acute suffering that occurs when people are denied family planning choices. At the same time, family planning differs from other branches of medicine in two critical ways: it is only successful when those concerned recognize that family planning involves consumer choices more than physician prescriptions and in most cases it deals with healthy people. It must be recognized that, although some contraceptives have been developed by medical researchers, the actual distribution of these methods, i.e. getting the right contraceptive to the right individual at the right place and right cost, involves many groups of service providers, the majority of them being non-clinical. The tension between consumer choices and conventional clinical perspectives is especially strong in the case of abortion. In putting this atlas together we have tried to keep these several perspectives in mind and, in order to better understand today's issues, we have also noted some of the history of family planning.

We are grateful to colleagues who have provided material and to the staff at Informa Healthcare for their patience and attention to detail. But above all we are grateful to the women and men all over the world who it has been our privilege to care for and who, in turn, have taught us the things we now know about this specialty. One thing we are certain about: family planning will continue to evolve and it will continue to remain important to hundreds of millions of people in all nations and of every background.

Pramilla Senanayake
Malcolm Potts

Acknowledgment

We would like to acknowledge Thusha Nawasiwatte, Dulani Siddhisena and Niraj Mahboob for the excellent research assistance they have provided during this project.

CHAPTER 1

Introduction

Reproduction is a lifelong process, not merely the passion of sexual intercourse or the pain of childbirth. It begins when the germ cells (which give rise to ova and sperm) are set aside early in embryonic life, and is still continuing when the grandparents do the babysitting. Medical science has been able to interrupt, or to devise potential new methods of contraception, at most steps in the long process from the formation of eggs and sperm to the fertilization of the egg, its attachment to the uterus, and the early embryonic development. Figure 1.1 shows the points in the process at which fertility can be controlled through intervention.

Family planning is wanted, simple, and inexpensive. It also involves areas of human sexuality which are perceived to be controversial and where public attitudes are conservative. The technologies which exist for the artificial control of human fertility need to be reviewed from two very different perspectives. The first is that of normal, healthy reproductive physiology; the second is that of public policy-making in an area of private concern.

Health professionals have a central role to play in family planning for two differing reasons. First, their work often gives them insight into private and intimate problems that

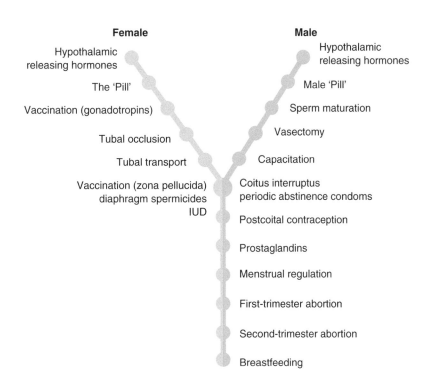

Female
Hypothalamic releasing hormones
The 'Pill'
Vaccination (gonadotropins)
Tubal occlusion
Tubal transport
Vaccination (zona pellucida) diaphragm spermicides
IUD

Male
Hypothalamic releasing hormones
Male 'Pill'
Sperm maturation
Vasectomy
Capacitation
Coitus interruptus periodic abstinence condoms
Postcoital contraception
Prostaglandins
Menstrual regulation
First-trimester abortion
Second-trimester abortion
Breastfeeding

Figure 1.1   The chart shows possible points of intervention to control fertility both up to and after the point of fertilization (not all the possibilities mentioned above are available in practice).

individuals may be reluctant to share with others; and, secondly, they have technical skills that are essential for the proper use of several – although by no means all – methods of fertility regulation.

It is easy to forget that human beings are the slowest breeding mammals known. Puberty occurs later than in any other species, and pregnancies are naturally spaced by long intervals of infertility associated with lactation. In addition, we are the only species with a clear-cut menopause followed by many years of infertile life in the female. In the few preliterate hunter–gatherer societies that are relatively untouched by the modern world, such as the !Khun from the Kalahari Desert or the Gangi from the highlands of New Guinea, puberty does not occur until the late teens or even early twenties. Babies are suckled on demand for 2 or 3 years and breastfeeding leads to the suppression of ovulation for 1–2 years. As a result, in the absence of any knowledge of contraception, pregnancies in preliterate societies are naturally spaced 3 or 4 years apart. Women in such societies commonly have only four to six live-born children in a lifetime; approximately half of these children die from childhood diseases and accidents before they themselves can reproduce. Thus, the population of the Kalahari !Khun doubles approximately every 300 years.

By contrast, in a modern society the age of puberty has fallen (probably as a result of nutritional changes). Patterns of breastfeeding have changed or the practice has been entirely replaced by bottle feeding: the technology of milk formula and prepared infant foods has had a remarkable effect on human fertility. In the absence of breastfeeding, a woman may have eight to ten live-born children in a lifetime. At the same time, a miraculous and welcome decline in infant mortality has occurred. The result: the population in a country such as contemporary Kenya doubles every 29 years. Worldwide, human beings now (2006) number 6.5 billion and the global population increases by 1 million every 4 days (Figure 1.2).

These changes have not only had a marked impact on potential family size but also they have had a catastrophically adverse effect on the health of individual women. Frequent childbearing, particularly amongst teenagers and women over the age of 35 years, greatly increases the risk of mortality and ill health among the women concerned. Less visible, but equally important, changes in the age of puberty (Figures 1.3 and 1.4) and in patterns of childbearing have

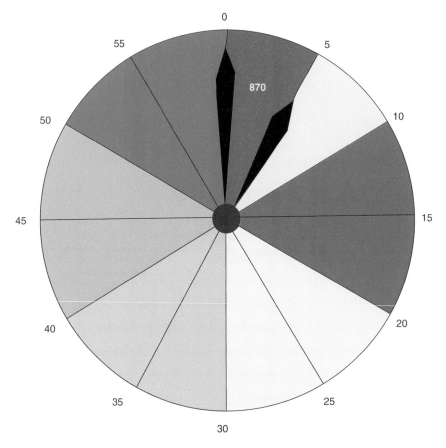

Figure 1.2 Rate of worldwide population increase. Worldwide, the population is increasing by 1 million every 4 days (i.e. by 870 every 5 minutes).

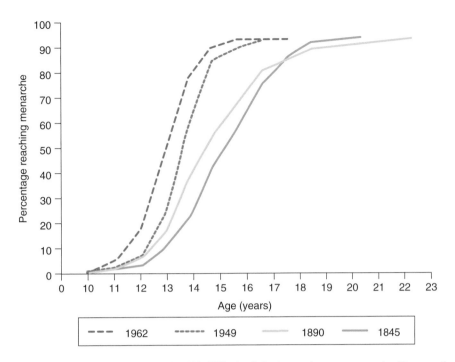

Figure 1.3 Changes in the age of menarche in England. In 1962, 50% of girls had started to menstruate by 13 years of age. A century earlier the corresponding figure was a little over 15 years. Also, as shown by the slope of the curve, the variation was greater in the 19th century, from 11 years to 19 years compared with 10–16 years for girls in the 1960s. (Adapted from reference 1.)

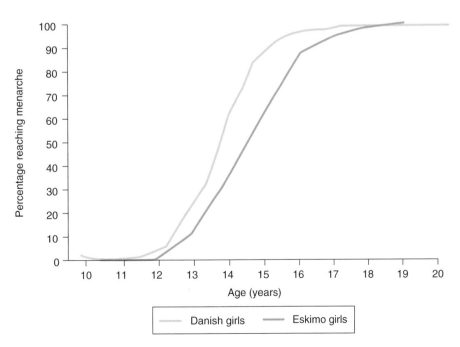

Figure 1.4 Age at menarche among the Eskimos in south-west Greenland compared with that of Danish girls in Copenhagen. Eskimo girls are about 2 years older than Danish ones at the stage when 50% are menstruating. (Adapted from reference 2.)

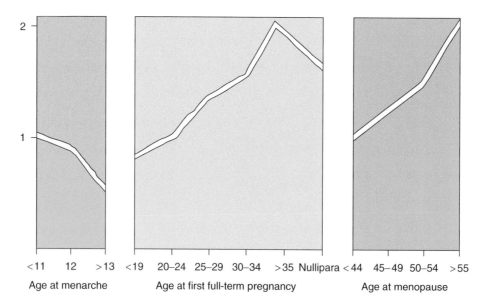

Figure 1.5 Relative risks for breast cancer.

been associated with an increased incidence of a number of diseases, particularly reproductive cancers. It is estimated that cancer of the breast is 120 times more common in Western women than in hunter–gatherer societies. Early menarche, late menopause, and late first full-term pregnancy are three risk factors for breast cancer (Figure 1.5).

REFERENCES

1. Parkes, AS. Patterns of Sexuality and Reproduction. Oxford: Oxford University Press, 1976: 18.
2. Parkes, AS. Patterns of Sexuality and Reproduction. Oxford: Oxford University Press, 1976: 19.

CHAPTER 2

Rationale for family planning

It is estimated that there are some 1.2 billion women of reproductive age in the world today. If on average each woman has two acts of intercourse per week this will amount to some 114 million acts of sexual intercourse taking place each day, resulting in 910 000 conceptions and 356 000 sexually transmitted bacterial and viral infections. There are more than 250 million new cases each year, at least one million of which will be HIV infection. Some developing-country family planning, antenatal, and maternal and child health clinics find that as many as one or two women in every 10 are infected with an STD.[1]

Reproduction in animals is characterized by a vast overproduction of sperm and eggs and a high degree of wastage of early pregnancy. A single human ejaculate represents more potential human beings than are found in the whole of the southern USA and Central America (Figure 2.1). A healthy man in his lifetime produces enough sperm to replace the whole human race.

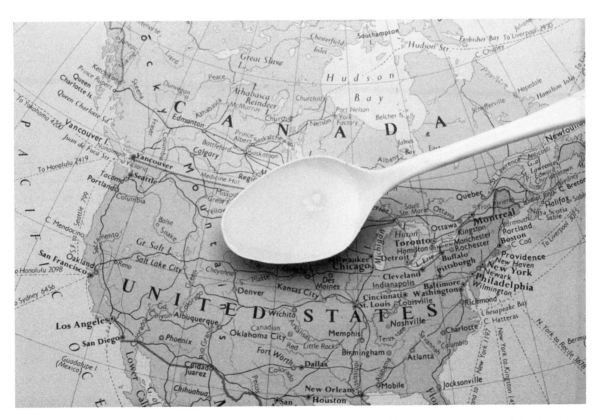

Figure 2.1   A single human ejaculate contained in this teaspoon represents more potential human beings than presently inhabit a large portion of North America. (Reproduced with kind permission from John Guillebaud.)

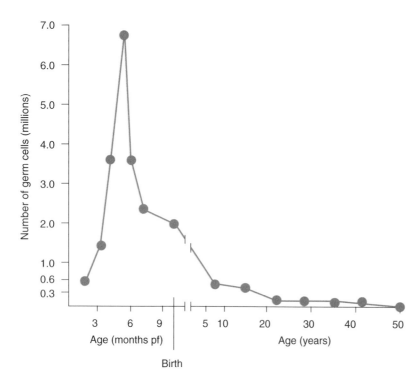

Figure 2.2 Numbers of germ cells in human ovaries (paired) from 2 months primordial follicles (pf) to menopausal age. (Adapted from reference 2)

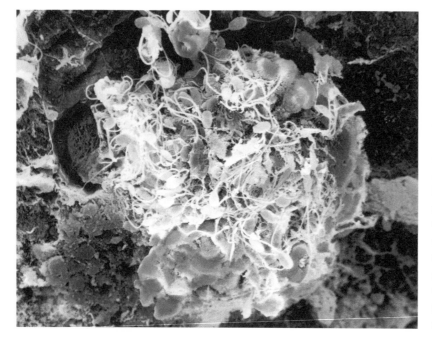

Figure 2.3 Fertilization: false-color scanning electron micrograph of a human egg almost surrounded by spermatozoa (blue). At the beginning of their journey in the vagina, the spermatozoa number about 300 million. The encounter between the egg and the few hundred surviving spermatozoa occurs in the ampullary region of the Fallopian tube. Only one spermatozoon may fertilize the egg and to do this it must penetrate a thick layer of follicular cells (pink) and the inner membrane known as the zona pellucida (not visible here). (Reproduced with kind permission from Professor P Motta, University of 'La Sapienza', Rome.)

Early in embryonic life a woman has over 6 million eggs, each genetically unique, in her ovaries. Most of these are lost before puberty; only a few hundred will be ovulated in her lifetime (Figure 2.2) and usually well under 20 will be fertilized (Figure 2.3). Many eggs and sperm have obvious microscopic defects and special studies show that chromosomal and other less visible abnormalities are even more common (Figures 2.4 and 2.5). Approximately half the eggs fertilized are naturally wasted even before a woman is aware that a pregnancy has taken place. Once a woman's period is late and pregnancy is recognized, up to 30% of embryos will still go on to abort spontaneously. The overwhelming majority of these early losses are of defective embryos that would not have survived to delivery, or if they did, would have produced grossly abnormal babies. Figure 2.6 illustrates the rate of spontaneous abortions by duration of pregnancy.

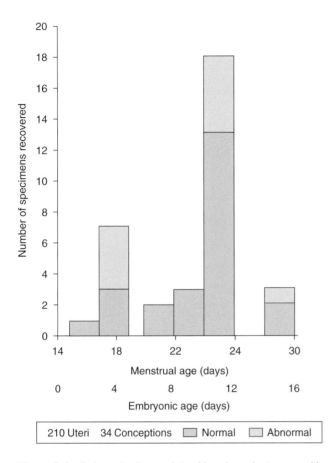

Figure 2.4 Embryonic abnormalities (thought to be incompatible with continuation of the pregnancy) detected prior to and shortly after the first missed period.

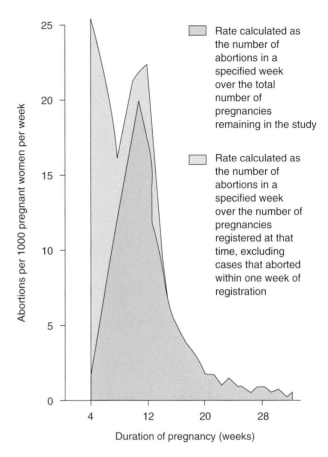

Figure 2.6 Spontaneous abortions by duration of pregnancy.

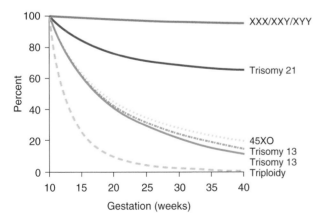

Figure 2.5 Gestational age-related risk for chromosomal abnormalities. The lines represent the relative risk according to the risk at 10 weeks of gestation. (From reference 4.)

In addition to this natural wastage, maternal and social factors contribute to the risk involved in any pregnancy. Family planning has a significant role to play in minimizing this risk for the individuals. At a cost of about $7.1 billion a year, modern contraceptive use currently prevents annually 187 million unintended pregnancies, 60 million unplanned births, 105 million

induced abortions, 2.7 million infant deaths, 215 000 pregnancy-related deaths, and 685 000 children losing their mothers due to pregnancy-related deaths.[5] In addition, the more people are helped to implement their personal choices about family size, the slower will be the growth in world population.

HEALTH RATIONALE

High-risk pregnancies

Birth planning can prevent high-risk pregnancies. The risk of maternal or infant morbidity and mortality is the highest in four specific types of pregnancies. In situations where maternal nutrition is not a problem, and where good and regular antenatal delivery and postnatal care are available, these risks may be somewhat reduced. The four high-risk groups are:

1. Too young – maternal age less than 18 years.
2. Too old – after age 35 years.
3. Too many – after four births.
4. Too close – less than 2 years apart.

Figure 2.7 shows how these factors interact.

Mothers too early

Globally, the percentage of women marrying under 20 years of age varies. It is estimated that 15 million girls aged 15–19 years give birth each year. Adolescent fertility rates are highest in developing regions such as south Asia and Sub-Saharan Africa (Table 2.1). Not surprisingly, the maternal mortality rates amongst women in this age group are also correspondingly highest in these areas (Figures 2.8 and 2.9).

This has both social (educational, emotional, and financial) and biological (prematurity, low birth weight, malnutrition, and infection) consequences. Adolescent mothers are at greater risk of pregnancy-induced hypertension and its complications, anemia, miscarriage, and obstetric complications (Figure 2.10). Their offspring are at increased risk of prematurity low birth weight, congenital abnormalities and, subsequently, higher infant mortality (Figure 2.11).

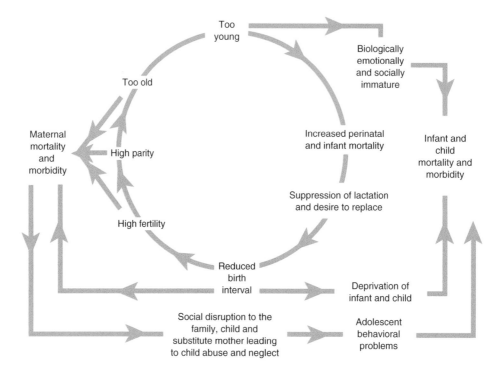

Figure 2.7 'Mothers too young, too old, too frequent, too many'; this scheme shows how these factors interact to increase the risk of maternal and infant mortality and morbidity.

Table 2.1   Adolescent fertility: Current status worldwide

UNICEF region	Annual number of births to girls aged 15–19 (millions) 2000–2005	Age-specific fertility rate (15–19 years) (annual births per 1000 girls aged 15–19) 2000–2005	Total fertility rate (2000) (lifetime births per woman at current fertility rates)
Sub-Saharan Africa	4.3	127	5.7
(Eastern/Southern Africa)	(1.9)	(111)	−5.5
(Western/Central Africa)	(2.4)	(143)	−5.9
Middle East/North Africa	0.7	39	3.7
South Asia	3.7	56	3.5
East Asia/Pacific	1.4	18	2
Latin America/Caribbean	1.8	71	2.6
Eastern Europe and former Soviet Union and Baltic States	0.7	35	1.6
Developing countries	12.8	Any	3
Least-developed countries	4.4	127	5.4
Industrialized countries	0.7	24	1.6
Total	13.4	50	2.7

From reference 6.

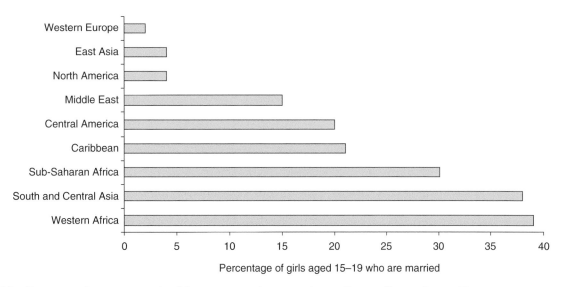

Figure 2.8 Percentage of women married in different countries/continents by age 19 years. (From reference 6.)

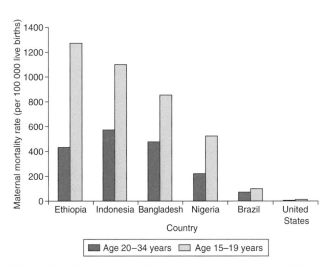

Figure 2.9 Maternal mortality is higher in younger women. (From references 7 and 8.)

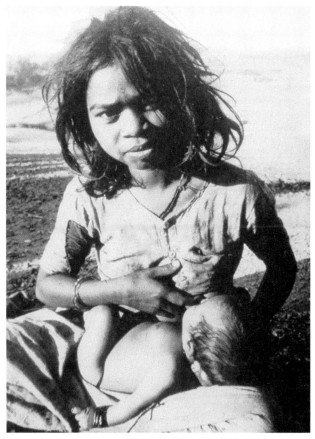

Figure 2.10 Malnourished 12-year-old mother and child. (From United Nations Population Fund.)

The child of multiple risks faces even greater problems. For example, a child born to a teenage mother less than 2 years after an earlier child faces an additional 116% risk of death before the age of 1 year if the previous child survived; if the previous child died, that additional risk rises to 320%.

Mothers too late

Late pregnancy also involves additional risk to mother and child. Studies have shown that advanced maternal age is associated with increased incidence of medical complications such as hypertension and diabetes, as well as obstetric complications. It is also well known that the incidence of Down's syndrome rises with advancing maternal age.

Recent evidence also suggests that it is not just the ovum which undergoes chromosomal changes with aging. After analyzing the sperm of more than 2000 men, a team

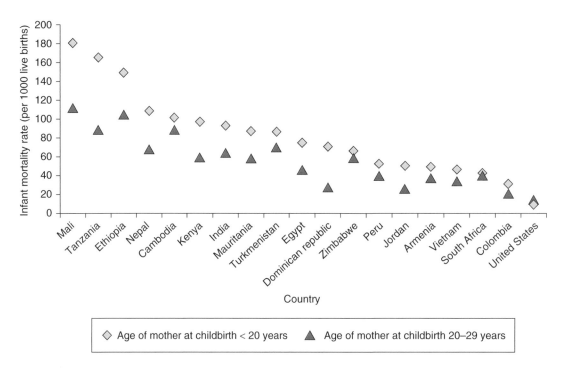

Figure 2.11   Infant mortality by age of mother: selected World Fertility Survey countries. (From reference 9.)

Table 2.2   Percentage of all births to women over 35 years of age

Country	Births to women over 35 years (%)
Uzbekistan	1.4
Romania	4.9
Portugal	14
Norway	15.2
Israel	15.6
Finland	18.9
Albania	8.3
Bulgaria	4.5

Data for 2001 from reference 11.

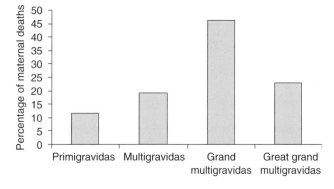

Figure 2.12   Maternal mortality rate by number of live births showing that maternal mortality increases with parity. (From reference 12.)

of scientists have found a wide and significant variation in the quality of sperm with advancing age. They claim that men over 45 years had double the amount of DNA damage compared with those younger than 30. Other parallel studies have confirmed this, and scientists hypothesize that as the sperm ages, it has more likelihood of being exposed to environmental toxins and oxidative stress, thus altering the genetic makeup, and rendering it possible for these mutations to be passed to the offspring of these men.[10]

Table 2.2 shows the percentage of all children born to women over 35 years of age in a number of countries.

Too many children

Were it not for the advent of contraception, a woman would bear around 12–15 children during her reproductive lifetime. In terms of risks and complications, the optimal number of children for a woman to bear is two or three. Pregnancies occurring after four births are associated with increased risks to both the mother and child (Figures 2.12 and 2.13). Serious complications of pregnancy and delivery including hemorrhage, infection, and eclampsia are more likely, as is anemia. The child faces the possibility of malnutrition due to increased family size, and is more likely to

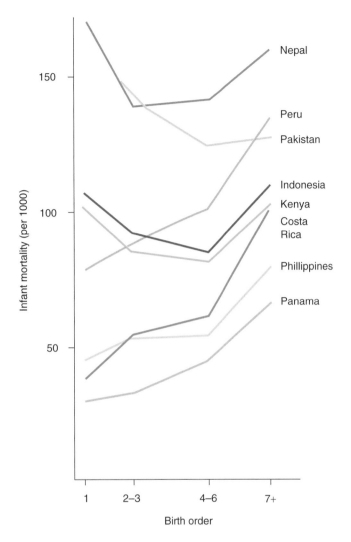

Figure 2.13 Infant mortality by birth order: selected World Fertility Survey countries. (From reference 13.)

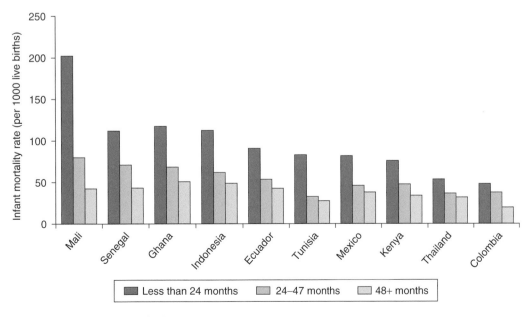

Figure 2.14 Birth spacing reduces infant deaths.

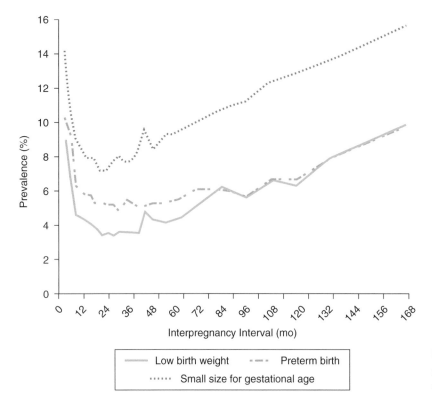

Figure 2.15 Effect of interval between pregnancies on perinatal outcome. From reference 14, with permission.

Table 2.3 Birth interval, measures of intelligence, and growth among 560 9-year-old children in Singapore. Results were independent of family size

Birth interval (months before index child)	Mean Mill Hill vocabulary scores	Mean Raven's Progressive Matrices scores	Mean heights (cm)	Mean weights (kg)	Teachers' assessments	
					Above average (%)	Below average (%)
<12	17.0	23.0	128.2	23.7	8.8	64.0
13–18	18.6	25.0	129.5	24.9	14.7	28.0
19–24	20.6	27.7	130.5	25.5	35.3	8.0
>24	20.9	28.2	131.7	26.3	41.2	0.0

From reference 15.

suffer from infectious illnesses, to have reduced physical growth and development, and less than optimal school performance.

Too close together

Pregnancies less than 2 years apart also pose increased risks to both mother and child. Frequent pregnancies cause a drain on the mother's nutritional status, and she may develop a maternal depletion syndrome. The child may have low birth weight and may suffer from malnutrition and poor health, as well as reduced physical growth and development, and decreased academic achievement. Figures 2.14 and 2.15 show the infant and child mortality rates according to spacing of pregnancies. Table 2.3 shows measures of intelligence and growth with respect to birth interval among children in Singapore.

As well as the increased likelihood of physical and intellectual problems, frequent births result in the mother devoting less time to each young child (Figure 2.16).

Maternal mortality/morbidity

Table 2.4 shows the estimated annual number of maternal deaths in various parts of the world. Maternal mortality rates vary from 2–160/100 000 live births in developed countries to 370–2000/100 000 in countries with low human development. In the USA, fewer than one of 100 deaths are of women in their child bearing years. This rises to one out of four deaths in developing countries. The causes of maternal mortality include obstetric factors, health service factors, low rates of contraceptive use and low socioeconomic status. Obstetric factors, which account for about two-thirds of all maternal deaths, include hemorrhage,

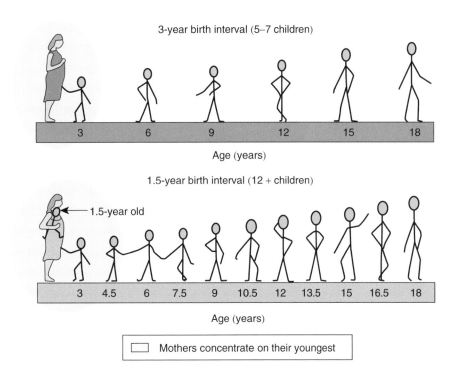

Figure 2.16 Diagrammatic representation of 'traditional' and 'modern' families, demonstrating differences in the amount of attention received by each child. With a 3-year birth interval (5–7 children), when the mother is 6 months pregnant, she has given her youngest 33 months' attention, which has to be shared with one other child. With a 1.5-year birth interval, when the mother is 6 months pregnant, she has given her youngest only 15 months' attention and this has to be shared with two other very young children.

Table 2.4 Maternal death statistics

Region	Maternal mortality ratio (maternal deaths per 1000 live births)	Number of maternal deaths	Lifetime risk of maternal death, 1 in:
World	400	529 000	74
Developed regions	20	2500	2800
Europe	24	1700	2400
Developing regions	440	527 000	61
Africa	830	251 000	20
Northern Africa	130	4600	210
Sub-Saharan Africa	920	247 000	16
Asia	330	253 000	94
Eastern Asia	55	11 000	840
South-Central Asia	520	207 000	46
South-Eastern Asia	210	25 000	140
Western Asia	190	9800	120
Latin America & the Caribbean	190	22 000	160
Oceania	240	530	83

From reference 16 with permission.

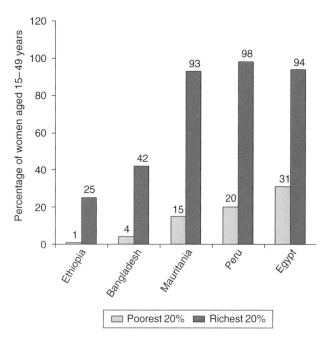

Figure 2.17 Births attended by skilled health personnel (doctor, nurse, or trained midwife) amongst the poorest and richest women in the country's population. (From reference 18, with permission.)

infection, pregnancy-induced hypertension and its complications, obstructed labor, and unsafe induced abortion. Health service factors which contribute to maternal mortality are lack of availability of treatment for complications, shortage of staff and supplies, and improper treatment (Figure 2.17).

Low rates of contraceptive use result in uncontrolled child-bearing, which in turn exposes high-risk women to the dangers of pregnancy. A woman's lifetime chance of maternal death accumulates, so that each pregnancy further increases the risk. Unwanted pregnancies prompt 'back street' abortions, which result in injury, sepsis, and various other complications leading to maternal deaths.

Low socioeconomic status often entails a lack of access to health care. In addition, malnutrition and a low social status of women contribute to maternal mortality.

A number of measures can be taken to reduce maternal mortality. Provision of family planning services, provision of obstetric first aid at health centers and rural maternity centers, upgrading of rural hospitals, expansion of the role of midwives, nurses, and medical assistants, establishment of maternity waiting homes, and community education are all of benefit in improving maternal health and reducing mortality. For example, Sri Lanka and Pakistan have the same gross national product, but the maternal mortality rate in Sri Lanka is one-tenth that of Pakistan; almost all births in Sri Lanka are attended by trained health personnel, and there are good family planning services and high female

literacy: Pakistan maternal mortality ratio (1985–2003), 530; Sri Lanka maternal mortality ratio (1990–2005), 43.

Child health problems related to high-risk pregnancy include low birth weight, prematurity, poor childhood nutrition, more frequent episodes of infectious diseases, slower physical growth and development, a higher risk of congenital abnormalities, and reduced intellectual performance. Anything which reduces a child's potential in life is an obscene thing – and lack of family planning is all too often just such a barrier to child development.

HUMAN RIGHTS/REPRODUCTIVE RIGHTS RATIONALE

Over the last 40 years or so the ability of individuals to choose the number and spacing of their children has been recognized as a basic human right. According to the World Population Plan of Action:[18] 'All individuals and couples have the right to decide freely and responsibly the number and spacing of their children and to have the information, education and the means to do so; the responsibility of couples and individuals in the exercise of this right takes into account the needs of their living and future children and their responsibilities towards the community'.

Individual world leaders and international meetings in Tehran (1968) and Mexico City (1984), as well as a number of declarations on human rights by the United Nations, and by Beijing (1995), all place an obligation on governments to offer their citizens family planning choices.

Unfortunately, a gap remains between political rhetoric and practical choices. Many individuals in the Third World simply do not have access to family planning information and services. Often, particular methods of family planning are not permitted or there are arbitrary limitations on access to voluntary surgical contraception and abortion.

The eroding status of low-income women in developing countries is a baseline indicator of human progress. Ignoring this issue is not only untenable; it is in the long run self-defeating. The health risks of poverty are far greater for females than for males. Policy measures for sustainable development must be accompanied by concrete actions towards the improvement of health, nutrition, sanitation, and access to safe water. In addition, effective family planning programs must be in place. If a woman is unable to control her fertility, it is unlikely that she will have control over the other aspects of her life.

DEVELOPMENT RATIONALE

For a thousand centuries following the evolution of our species, parents, on average, could expect to see two children survive and reproduce in the next generation, even though

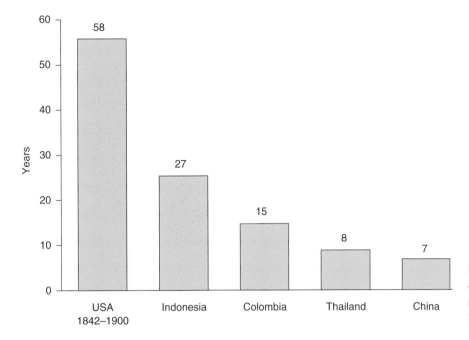

Figure 2.18 Fertility trends in selected countries (expressed as the number of years it took for family size to fall from 6.0 to 3.5). (From reference 20.)

they might have delivered four to six babies. If this was not true, the 'population explosion' would have happened a long time ago. Then, for about 100 years in the West and 50 years in the developing world, a rapid fall in infant mortality and changes in breastfeeding patterns that increased fertility suddenly meant that four to six children were surviving until the next generation. As a result, the global population has doubled at shorter and shorter intervals.

According to the US National Academy of Sciences 1986 Report,[19] the world as a whole is in transition. Fertility has fallen to 48% of the birth rates found after the Second World War to family sizes which would be compatible with a stable global population. In some developing countries where good family planning services have been made available, the birth rate has fallen two to four times as rapidly as it did in the West at a similar stage of the demographic transition (Figure 2.18).

The declining fertility in Western Europe and North America in the 19th and 20th centuries was almost certainly seriously retarded by lack of access to contraceptive choices. Hospital records for women admitted for complications of illegal abortion in the first half of the 20th century are a testimony to the innumerable desperate attempts made by women to restrict family size.

There is a consistent relationship between the birth rate and the use of contraceptives. For every 15% rise in contraceptive prevalence, the average number of children in a family falls by one. Wherever contraceptives have been readily available, and particularly where safe abortion services have been accessible, fertility has fallen rapidly. There was a time when demographers argued that there were

intrinsic differences in desired family size between various social, economic, and religious groups. In practice, wherever the barriers to fertility regulation have been removed, differences in various groups have disappeared. This is well illustrated by the history of Protestant and Catholic groups in the USA since 1950: for a while, Catholic fertility was consistently higher than Protestant, but once contraceptives became acceptable and widely available and abortion was legalized, the differences disappeared. Interestingly, there is little or no difference in the percentage of women of different religious groups who resort to abortion (Figure 2.19).

THE POPULATION EXPLOSION

How long will it take for the second half of the global demographic transition to be completed? Until approximately 10 000 years ago, the world population was no more than 5 million. The transition from hunting–gathering to settled agriculture meant that many more people could be supported by the same area of land. The result was a gradual increase in the population, which reached about 200 million by the time of Christ. By 1987, the world population had exceeded 5 billion. This landmark shows the unprecedented rate of growth of the human population. The first billion was not reached until 1830. It then took 100 years to reach the second billion, but only 45 years to double again to 4 billion in 1975. The 6 billion mark was surpassed 25 years later in the year 2000, and the current population has bordered upon 6.5 billion (Figure 2.20). The fact that the world is in a demographic transition means exactly that; in most communities there are some people

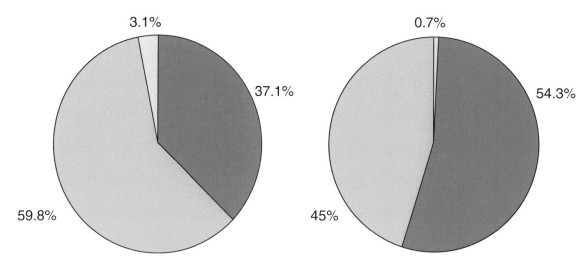

Figure 2.19 The percentage of Protestants, Catholics, and other religious groups in the canton and city of Basle, 1960 (left), and the percentage of women from these populations having abortions (n=320) (right). Protestant, yellow; Catholic, blue; other religious groups, pink

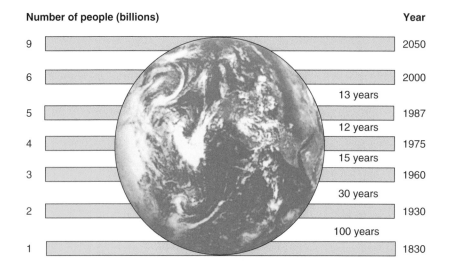

Figure 2.20 The United Nations prediction. The pattern of population increase up to 2050, and the number of years required to add one billion more people.

who, sufficiently desperate to control their fertility, will resort to abortion, while there are others who adhere to traditional ways and continue to want large families of four to eight children. Fertility is lower in urban areas where incomes are high, where education is prevalent, where the status of women is high, and where women go out to work. However, these are correlates of fertility, not causes. Fertility declines only when people abstain from sex, use contraceptives effectively, or have abortions.

In every developing country for which data are available, there is a measurable unmet need for family planning, and people's achieved family sizes exceed their desires. This is not to say that everyone wants to adopt contraceptive methods immediately, but it should direct programming towards increasing the availability of safe, effective, and inexpensive methods of contraception and abortion. In broad terms,

particularly where government and private medical services are few and far between and overburdened with aspects of curative medicine, this means making oral contraceptives, injectables, and condoms available through simple channels; this usually involves their subsidized sale through existing commercial outlets, drawing the doctors back to the provision of voluntary surgical contraception, and dealing with the public health issues associated with abortion.

The 21st century

The world has within its grasp a remarkable opportunity. A great deal has been learned about family planning in the first half of the demographic transition: it is a simple, cheap, wanted set of choices that are well understood and that give predictable results. Use has been held back by shortage of resources, restrictive medical practices, confused public policies,

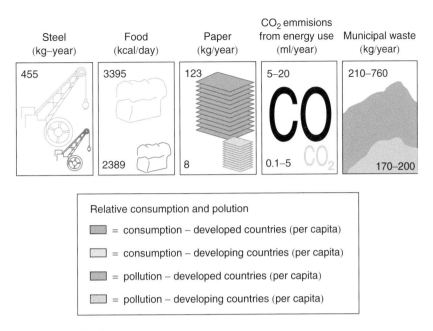

Figure 2.21   Relative consumption and pollution.

and general lack of realism. The challenge before the world is to learn from past experience and accomplish the second half of the demographic transition more rapidly. The rate of global population growth has fallen marginally, but absolute numbers continue to rise. By chance, the annual growth in global population has been approximately in step with the calendar year: 95 million more births than deaths in 1995, 96 million in 1996 and so on until the end of the decade. More babies were born in the last decade of the 20th century than in any other 10 years in human history. If the present unmet need for contraception could be satisfied, maternal mortality could easily be reduced by 25–35%.

As a result of yesterday's population explosion, there are one-sixth more women of fertile age in the year 2005 than there were a decade ago. If contraceptive prevalence continues to rise and more women are to be served, then, as a rule of thumb, it may well be possible to double the number of contraceptive users in the present decade.

Some time between now and the year 2010, a year will dawn when there will be fewer babies born than in the year before. The date of this inflexion in the growth of the human population will largely predict the final level of the population of the world. In fact, the USA has already claimed this achievement, as statistics have shown that the birth rate in the USA was lower in 2002 than in any year since records going back to the late 19th century. A recent survey by the United Nations predicted that the world population would stabilize at 9 million, by the year 2300. Nevertheless, the same report warns that if the current rate of global population growth prevailed, and family planning continued to receive the low priority it has been given by the international

community in the past, the world population would continue to increase to an incredible and unsustainable level of 1.34 trillion by year 2300! Affluent Westerners consume much more of the world's resources and pollute much more of its environment than Third World rice farmers or the underemployed or unemployed of Third World urban slums (Figure 2.21). Developmental assistance and political systems are predicated, however, on the principle that poor people will get richer.

Human numbers are already challenging the ability of the biosphere to accommodate the human race. Global grain reserves are getting less, the environment is changing, global warming may have begun, the holes in the ozone layer are enlarging, tropical forests are disappearing, the Sahara is spreading, large areas of the ocean are polluted, and fish yields are falling in many places. Even if these problems can be overcome, finding the capital and job opportunities to employ ever-increasing numbers of young people is an almost impossible challenge.

Some time in the next 100 years the world has to complete the transition from the present energy-intensive industrial societies and intensive agriculture, to a biologically sustainable set of systems. We must move from an economy dependent on fossil fuels and other non-renewable resources to a biologically sustainable economy where we take no more from the environment than living processes can renew, and put no more back into the environment as pollution than the living processes can absorb. This most challenging of transitions must be accomplished while the world also attempts to lift increasingly large numbers of people out of abysmal poverty to some semblance of dignity and freedom from poverty. It may well prove the most technically difficult task the human race has faced. Science can solve many problems and Cassandras have been proved wrong in the past. But as we press at the finite limits of the planet we must remind ourselves that every problem must be overcome or irreversible damage will be done at least to parts of our environment.

The final stable population of the world will be a key factor determining success or failure in this ultimate test of political, technical, and economic systems. A world of 10 billion people, even given goodwill and luck – which are not always abundantly available – will find it difficult to adjust to twice its present population, particularly as many of these people will be consuming much more than they do at present. A world with three times as many people might well fail to make the adjustment.

The sight of a few tens or hundreds of thousands of people dying of starvation in the horn of Africa or swept into the sea by cyclones in Bangladesh is deeply disturbing. A world where, in order to balance human numbers, a million people might die every 4 days is an unthinkable horror.

People want smaller families, and family planning is well understood and cheap to make available. Our children and grandchildren will never forgive today's leaders if we do not take the opportunity for making family planning universally available in the near future. The costs would be trivial: the cost of inaction immeasurable (Figure 2.22).

In parts of Europe (e.g. Germany and Italy) the average family size has fallen below two children – that is, the population is imploding. In the developing world, in every country that has been surveyed, women want fewer children

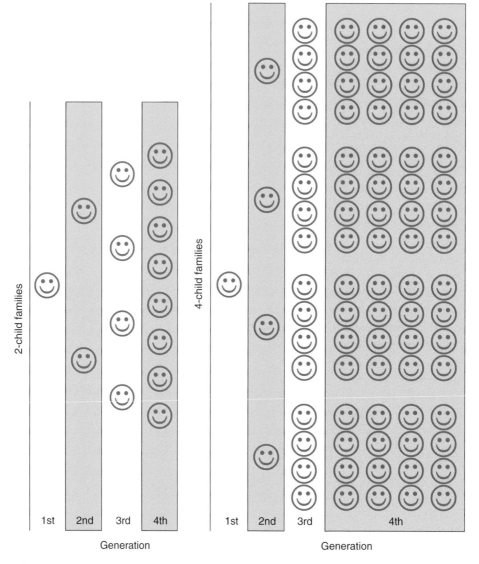

Figure 2.22 Bigger families, faster population growth. Four generations of 2- and 4-child families.

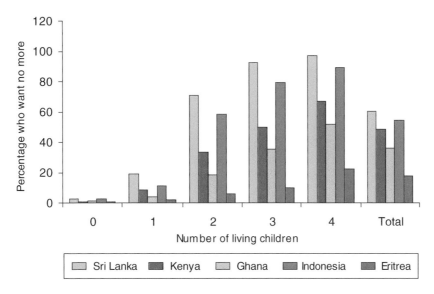

Figure 2.23   Desire to stop childbearing amongst currently married women, by number of living children. (From reference 5.)

than they are having, and wherever there are data available, the proportion of women not wanting any more children has risen in the past 10 years (Figure 2.23).

There is little or no evidence that Americans want fewer or smaller cars, Indians fewer refrigerators, Scandinavians fewer flights to winter holidays in the sun; or that any of a million other demands for energy and raw materials, or the production of greenhouse gases or ozone-destroying chemicals will decline quickly. People all over the planet want smaller families; failure to respond to that need not only condemns millions of women to suffer the misery of unintended pregnancy – and even death from abortion – but also may well prove the deciding factor in the long-term survival of the fragile ecosystem that is the only home the human family has known or may ever know.

REFERENCES

1. Populations Reports volume xxi, No 1 June 1993.
2. Baker TG. A quantitative and cytological study of germ cells in human ovaries. Proc R Soc Lond B Biol Sci 1963; 158: 417–33.
3. http://www.bbc.co.uk/health/awareness_campaigns/feb_contraceptive.shtml
4. Nicolaides KH, Sebire NJ, Snijders RJM, Souka AP. Calculation of risk for chromosomal defects. In: Nicolaides KH, Sebire NJ, Snijders RJM, Souka AP, eds. The 11–14-Week Scan. Carnforth, UK: Parthenon Publishing, 1999: 7–14.
5. State of the World Population Report, The Cairo consensus at Ten: Population, Reproductive Health, and the Global effort to end poverty. New York UNFPA 2004.
6. UN population Division. Population Estimates and projections 2000 Revision. In UNICEF statistics – Fertility & contraceptive use.
7. The Safe motherhood & Action Agenda; Priorities for the next decade. Report on the safe motherhood, Technical consultation 18-23 October 1997 Colombo, Sri Lanka. New York Family Care International 1998.
8. Centers for Disease Control and Prevention, 2002.
9. DHS data since 1990; Centers for Disease Control and Prevention, 2002.
10. Sikka SC. Oxidative stress and role of antioxidants in normal and abnormal sperm function. Front Biosci 1996; 1: e78–86.
11. Trends in Europe and North America 2005. The Statistical Pocketbook of the Economic Commission for Europe. UN Economic Commission, 2005.
12. Begum S, Aziz-un-Nisa, Begum I. Analysis of maternal mortality in a tertiary care hospital to determine causes and preventable factors. J Ayud Med Coll Abbottabad 2003; 15: 49–52.
13. Acsadi GTF, Johnson-Acsadi G. Family Planning and Well-Being of Women and Children. London: IPPF, 1985.
14. Zhu BP, Rolfs RT, Nangle E, Horan JM. Effect of the interval between pregnancies on perinatal outcomes. N Engl J Med 1999; 340: 589–94.
15. Martin CE. J Trop Paediatr 1978; 25: 45–76.
16. Maternal mortality in 2000: estimates developed by WHO, UNICEF, and UNFPA.
17. World Bank. Round II Country Reports on Health, Nutrition, and Population Conditions Among the Poor and Better-off in 56 Countries. World Bank, 2004.
18. World Population Plan of Action. Mexico City, 1984.
19. US National Academy of Sciences 1986 Report. Population Growth and Economic Development: Policy Questions.
20. United Nations Population Fund. The State of World Population, 1991. New York: United Nations Population Fund, 1991.

CHAPTER 3

History of family planning

The history of family planning is the history of conflict between the majority of the community, who are often vividly aware of the socioeconomic need to restrain fertility, and social elites, who, although they are the first to restrict the size of their own families, tend to maintain the political, legal, and ecclesiastical status quo. Conservative attitudes have influenced the rate at which various technologies affecting human fertility have been developed and have diffused throughout society. For example, there were no political, legal, or theological comments on the introduction of either wet nursing in the 16th and 17th centuries or artificial milk formulae in the late 19th and 20th centuries but, by contrast, a great deal of controversy has surrounded the availability of contraceptives and the choices of voluntary surgical contraception and abortion.

The use of coitus interruptus to control fertility is referred to in the Bible and simple barrier methods of contraception are known from ancient Egypt. The history of modern family planning began in the early 19th century with the writings of Francis Place, Robert Dale Owen, and John Stuart Mill, in Britain, along with Charles Knowlton in the USA. Society tends to be conservative in most matters of reproduction and it is significant that these early leaders were free thinkers, who rejected contemporary religion.

The Christian rejection of birth control reached its most forceful expression in the writings of Saint Augustine (354–430) and Saint Thomas Aquinas (1225–74). Augustine argued that original sin was an entity transmitted in the semen, rather like a latter day AIDS virus. In the Bible (*Genesis* 38:9), Onan 'when he went into his (dead) brother's wife ... he emitted on the ground, lest he should give an heir to his brother. And the thing which he did displeased the Lord: wherefore he slew him.' Theologians are divided as to whether Onan's sin was to practice coitus interruptus or to disobey his father and not raise children by his dead brother's wife. Be that as it may, Augustine interpreted

all forms of contraception as anathema. For a millennium and a half the Catholic Church taught that contraception was a sin, in some cases worse than adultery or abortion.

The conflict between orthodox religion and family planning grew during the nineteenth century and has continued to this day. In 1877, Charles Bradlaugh and Annie Besant republished Charles Knowlton's book *The Fruits of Philosophy* (1832). Knowlton had described coitus interruptus, albeit in coy terms; on republication Bradlaugh and Besant were tried and convicted under the Obscene Publications Act, but subsequently acquitted on a technicality. The publicity associated with the trial put contraception 'onto the breakfast tables' of the English middle classes and from 1877 onwards the birth rate in Britain began to decline. In 1873 the United States went in the opposite direction when Anthony Comstock persuaded Congress that anything to do with contraception was an obscenity and that birth control information should not be distributed through the postal system.

In Britain the opposition to family planning was less extreme than in the USA, but almost as destructive; by 1910 15% of English couples had used contraception at some time during their marriage and by 1935–39, two-thirds. But religious teaching remained at variance with the conscience of the flock until the 1920 Lambeth Conference when the Anglican Church cautiously accepted family planning. Catholic teaching continues to reject family planning and in 1968 Pope Paul issued the encyclical *Humanae Vitae*, excluding all methods of contraception except for periodic abstinence. Paradoxically, this was one method which Saint Augustine had specifically and explicitly condemned.

Margaret Sanger (Figure 3.1) was a public health nurse practicing in New York. One of the women she cared for, Sadie Sachs, was recovering from an illegal abortion. Mrs Sanger asked the doctor how Mrs Sachs might prevent

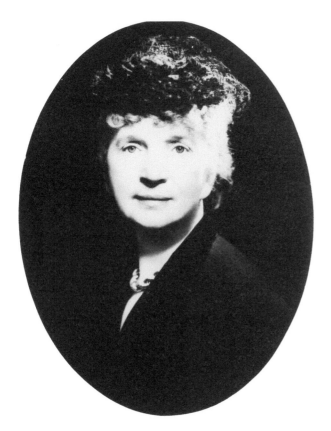

Figure 3.1 Margaret Sanger, an early US family planning crusader, opened the first family planning clinic in America in 1916 but was indicted and imprisoned for her efforts.

further pregnancies and he flippantly replied that Sadie's husband should 'sleep on the roof'. When Sadie had a second abortion and died, Margaret Sanger was propelled into a life-long crusade for family planning. She published a million copies of her *Family Limitation*. She visited Europe to learn about Mensinga's diaphragm and opened the first family planning clinic in America in Brooklyn in 1916. Under the Comstock laws she was indicted and imprisoned (Figure 3.2).

Eventually, the Comstock laws were interpreted so as to permit qualified medical personnel to give contraceptive advice 'for the cure and prevention of disease'. In 1936, in the celebrated case known as 'The United States vs One Package', Mr Justice Hand further modified the Comstock Acts so as to permit 'the importation, sale or carriage by mail of things that might intelligently be employed by conscientious and competent physicians for the purpose of saving life or promoting the well-being of their patients'. The Comstock Acts themselves, however, were not finally struck down until the Supreme Court case of Griswald vs Connecticut in 1965.

FERTILITY CONTROL – A HISTORY OF CONFLICT

Although fertility control, as noted, has had an important impact on the health of women and children, it is not a therapy

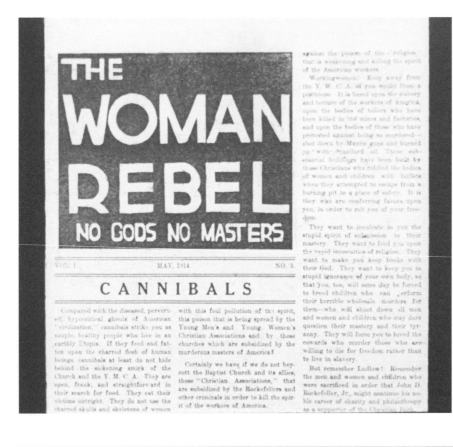

Figure 3.2 The Woman Rebel: No Gods, No Masters', Margaret Sanger's case, as reported in the media.

prescribed to control diseases but a series of choices that informed individuals make. The conflict between private choice and public conservatism, and between science and religion in the field of fertility control has found its expression in the long, acrimonious, and still destructive collision between those who would restrict access to family planning or who see it as a series of therapies to be prescribed, and those who see all restrictions as unnecessary and believe that adults have a basic human right to choose from or reject the variety of technologies that now exist to control fertility.

This conflict restrains and confuses the medical profession in three overlapping ways. First, for good reasons, the practice of medicine tends to be conservative and this conservatism is transmitted to the rest of society who look to the medical profession for leadership in anything to do with the human body or the health of the family. Secondly, the perceived need of society to make family planning 'respectable', as is exemplified by the USA vs One Package, when physicians became the fig leaves society needed to douse legal or political controversy. Unfortunately, it is a policy that also makes contraception more difficult to obtain and thrusts doctors into a controlling position in family planning even when they were not clinically relevant. In 2004, the US Food and Drug Administration (FDA) overrode its scientific advisers and blocked their recommendation to permit over-the-counter sale of emergency contraception in the USA.[1]

Thirdly, public controversy over family planning retarded scientific investigation. The US National Institutes of Health, the world's largest funder of medical research, were held back by Congress legislation from working in family planning until 1960. Between the two World Wars research

into spermicides by Dr JR Baker at Oxford University led to him being thrown out his laboratory; Dr Baker was only rescued by Professor Howard Florey, later the Nobel Prize winner for the development of penicillin. In the World Health Assembly, the Vatican State prevented the World Health Organization responding to requests for assistance from developing countries in family planning until 1965. The conflict has not abated in the 21st century as the Bush administration in America has attempted to impose a conservative agenda on international agencies and meetings involved in family planning and decisions by the FDA and information disseminated by the Centers for Disease Control (CDC) have become politicized.

Be brave and angry

Pioneers of family planning in the West in the 19th and early 20th centuries and more recent leaders in the developing countries have a great deal in common. Despite the efforts of the early campaigners, family planning is still not without obstacles, even in developed countries. In 1990–91, the Irish Family Planning Association was prosecuted in Dublin for selling condoms in the Virgin Music Megastore. Disputes over abortion legislation almost stalled the reunification of Germany and, in 1993, Poland reversed a previously liberal abortion law.

In Iran in February 1979, the former president of the Family Planning Association was almost executed 'for the killing of 5000 infants' – this being the misinterpretation of young religious fundamentalists of 5000 women who had used her clinics. Fortunately, however, Islam is the only one of the world's great religions to teach a positive message about family planning (providing a man has his wife's consent to

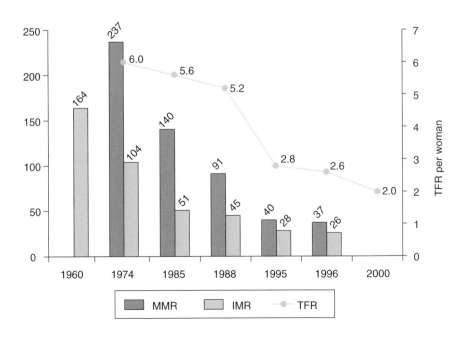

Figure 3.3 While Iranian fundamentalists attacked family planning in the 1970s, by the late 1980s the religious leadership had endorsed family planning ('for the woman's health') and once contraception and voluntary sterilization were made available the birth rate fell as rapidly as it had in China, but without a one child policy. MMR, maternal mortality; IMR, infant mortality, TFR, total fertility rate (Source: Ministry of Health and Medical Education, Iran.)

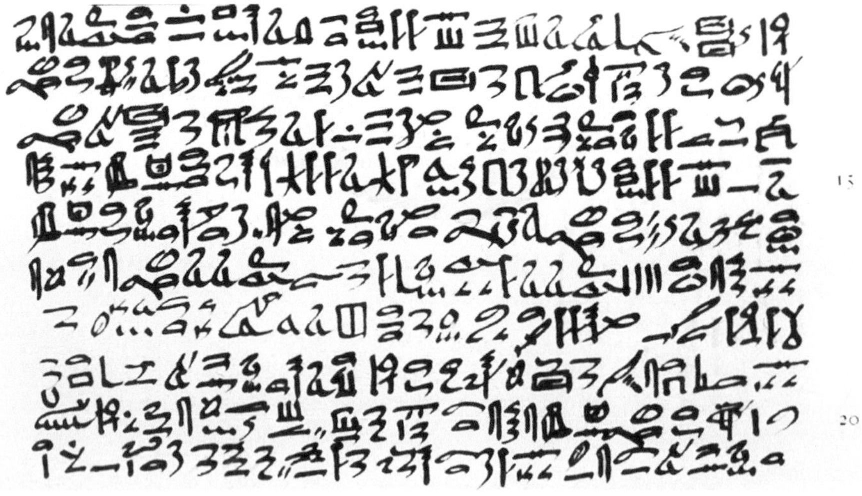

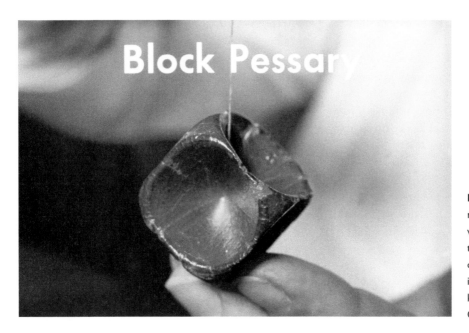

Figure 3.4 The *Ebers* papyrus dates back to 1550 BC and recommends a medicated tampon designed 'to cause that a woman should cease to conceive for 1, 2, or 3 years'. The ingredients include seedwool moistened with honey, ground acacia, and dates. (Courtesy of the IPPF.)

Block Pessary

Figure 3.5 One of the most unusual barrier methods was the block pessary which was inserted into the vagina in the hope that one of the concave surfaces would fit over the cervix. It was described as an instrument of torture. (Reproduced with kind permission from Ortho-McNeil Inc., Canada.)

practice contraception). In the 1990s the Islam Republic of Iran made family planning widely available and family size plummeted from almost six children to replacement level. At the same time, and partly as a consequence of this dramatic change in family size, infant and maternal mortality fell (Figure 3.3) and the percentage of women in Iranian universities overtook men.

HISTORY OF CONTRACEPTION

Fertility can be restored to lower levels by the use of contraception, by resort to abortion, or a combination of the two. Efforts to control human fertility are as old as written history.

Medical papyri from Egypt (Figure 3.4) describe contraceptive suppositories including one based on crocodile dung! In their efforts to prevent or abort pregnancy, women have ingested a huge variety of concoctions. Some have been poisonous, such as ergot, or useless, such as dried beaver testicles (a brew once drunk by Canadian native peoples). Other traditional remedies may have helped, such as contraceptive sponges dipped in vinegar or lime/lemon juice and placed against the cervix. In the 18th century, Casanova advocated using a half lemon from which the juice had been extracted as a cervical cap. The block pessary gained a bad reputation due to its awkward shape; in 1931 it was considered more an instrument of torture than a prevention of pregnancy (Figure 3.5). The

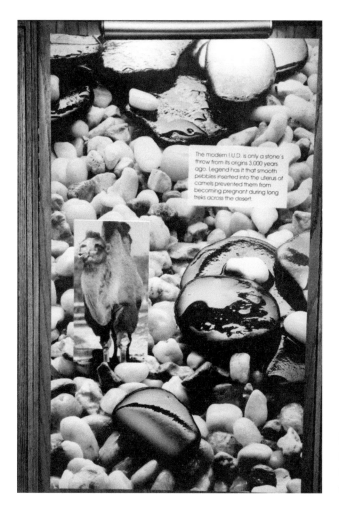

The modern I.U.D. is only a stone's throw from its origins 3,000 years ago. Legend has it that smooth pebbles inserted into the uterus of camels prevented them from becoming pregnant during long treks across the desert.

Figure 3.6 The modern intrauterine device (IUD) may have originated from the practice of placing smooth pebbles in the uterus of a camel to prevent it from becoming pregnant during long treks across the desert. (Courtesy of the IPPF.)

modern intrauterine device (IUD) is only a stone's throw from its origins 3000 years ago; legend has it that smooth pebbles inserted into the uteri of camels prevented them from becoming pregnant during long treks across the desert (Figure 3.6). Today's intrauterine devices owe their designs to the wishbone intracervical pessaries and stem plugs of the early 1900s. Some wishbones were fashioned from 10 and 14 carat gold, and sometimes stem plugs were sutured to the uterus wall to prevent expulsion (see Figure 9.1).

Birth control methods have come a long way since the concoctions prescribed in the *Ebers* papyrus, but the perfect contraceptive still remains elusive. Researchers are continually exploring new methods, such as long-acting subdermal implants, contraceptive patches, and male oral contraceptives (see Chapter 15).

REFERENCE

1. https//www.npr.org/templates/story/story.php?storyId=1875868

CHAPTER 4

Human sexuality, including female reproduction and male physiology

SEX AND REPRODUCTION

It is usual to begin by describing the anatomy and physiology of human reproduction; however, these attributes can be understood only in a broader context of human sexual behavior.

The human species, like other animals, is judged by evolution according to the number of its offspring that survive to the next generation and reproduce. The male (Figure 4.1) and female anatomies and reproductive physiology and behavior have been tailored over millions of years of evolution to provide for the optimal performance. As a viviparous animal that usually bears one young alive at a time, after a long interval of pregnancy and before an even longer interval of lactation, the anatomy, physiology, and behavior of the two sexes are very different: the woman provides a disproportionate share of the energy and time which must be devoted to reproducing the next generation. A woman can only conceive, feed, and care for a relatively small number of children in her relatively brief fertile life, while a man, if he is ruthless and competitive, can father a relatively large number of children.

The size of the testicles and the number of sperm produced by men, in relative terms, are less than those among chimpanzees, who are highly promiscuous in their mating, but more than in truly monogamous primates, such as the Marmoset monkey. Men make enough sperm for intercourse a few times a week, rather than perhaps several times a day, as do chimpanzees.

BRAIN AND BEHAVIOR

The primary and largest sex organ in the human species is above the waist – the brain. It has been plausibly argued that every aspect of other systems (the locomotive system, nervous

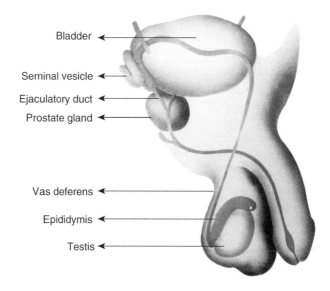

Figure 4.1   Male reproductive anatomy

system, etc.) has been driven in evolution by the need to reproduce. The very large brain that characterizes our species, and enables us to read and write books, may have evolved as a result of sexual competition within our own species. After all, some animals with very small brains, such as the dinosaurs, lived on this earth much longer than the human species is likely to survive, and others, such as rats, exploit almost as many different environments as we do. Once an animal evolves a certain proficiency in finding its food, then competition in reproduction comes not from the outside world but from other members of the species and even of the same sex. Possibly our big brains evolved so that we can manipulate one another in the endless competition to secure a mate and to build the bonds between the sexes which are essential to bring up a baby whose brain is so large that it endangers the life of the mother during delivery and who requires continuous close attention for many years during its own development.

The other large apes to whom we are so closely related (human beings and chimpanzees have 98% of their DNA in common) are either polygamous (as is the gorilla) or promiscuous (as are chimpanzees). The males compete with one another for access to the females and, although they may guard the territory from which the females draw their food supply, they play no role in bringing up the next generation.

At some point in relatively recent evolution, the human newborn achieved a threshold size of brain, becoming so totally dependent for so long an interval of time that it was in the biological interest of both sexes to work together to nurture their offspring. In all human societies (although to varying degrees), males accept paternity for their children and make a direct contribution to their upbringing. The key event in the evolution of human sexual behavior, that made the change from a promiscuous primate, like a chimpanzee, to the partially monogamous mating system found in humankind, was the concealment of ovulation in the female.

Human beings are alone among other species in that ovulation in women is not associated with the prominent physical changes seen in other primates (such as the vivid vulval swellings of chimpanzees or baboons), or the behavior changes of estrus seen in other mammals (such as the domestic cat). Even though human pheromones do exist, they are not sufficiently powerful to be detected by males as compared with the pheromones in most animal species. Physical changes associated with ovulation, such as midcycle pain in some women, changes in cervical mucus consistency, rise in body temperature, etc, are often subtle and rarely recognized by the woman herself. Men and women can have sexual intercourse on any day of the menstrual cycle, during much of pregnancy, lactation, and after the menopause. Humans do not depend on an 'estrus' to be physically attracted to each other, and unlike in many animal species, the female does not lose interest in the male when her period of 'heat', or ovulation, is over. Two things follow from this unusual form of behavior. First, the male mating strategy has switched from coitus with any available ovulating female, towards establishing a long-term relationship with one woman – a relationship of love founded on sexual desire and passion. But, a state bordering on perpetual sexual arousal and receptivity, among the adults of an intensely social animal (which we most obviously are), also brings in its wake some secondary problems.

Evolution appears to have built in some additional behaviors to prevent our species falling into sexual chaos: again, if we think of how other animals behave, we are the only species where adults, in all known societies, cover their genitals in public, and all adults in all known societies normally make love in private, commonly after dark and usually isolated from other members of their social group.

Behavior leaves no fossil record and it is impossible to be certain by which specific steps our mating system evolved from our *Australopithicene* ancestors, but concealed ovulation, secret copulation, and covering our external genitalia – even totally naked aboriginal tribes in Australia used to stand back to back and talk to one another when adults from different clans met – are unique behavioral strategies that appeared relatively recently in our evolution and are the basis of the human mating system. They are also probably the key to understanding the need for, and the politics of, family planning: most episodes of sexual intercourse are manifestly not for procreation, but to reinforce the bond of sexual love between parents; and yet we are all shy about sex and, just as we cover our external sex organs in public, so we – not unnaturally – find discussion of sex difficult, and often make mistakes in establishing public policies relating to reproduction.

ENDOCRINE CONTROL

Both men and women produce the same set of pituitary and gonadal hormones. In women, libido is also thought to depend on circulating testosterone. However, the pituitary control of follicle-stimulating hormone (FSH) and luteinizing hormone (LH) in the two sexes differs.

The male secondary sexual characteristics and sexual behavior are primarily driven by testosterone, although there is no close correlation between the frequency of intercourse and testosterone levels, and neither has any consistent difference in male physiology been discovered in the case of men who choose a homosexual lifestyle.

Modern civilized living has brought about relatively few changes in the way that men use their reproductive systems – other than an important decline in the age of the onset of puberty. But in women, modern living brings about profound changes, with important life-long consequences.

Many textbooks on medicine look upon the 28-day menstrual cycle as a normal situation for a healthy adult woman. In reality, the reproductive system was evolved to do just that – to reproduce. When healthy women have unprotected intercourse, about one-third of them become pregnant in the first cycle and the majority after three or four cycles. The natural situation is for FSH and LH to control ovulation, and then for FSH and LH produced by the fertilized egg to block the disruption of the endometrium. If conception does not take place, the endometrium is shed; the embryo and fetus have 'highjacked' the female reproductive system (Figure 4.2).

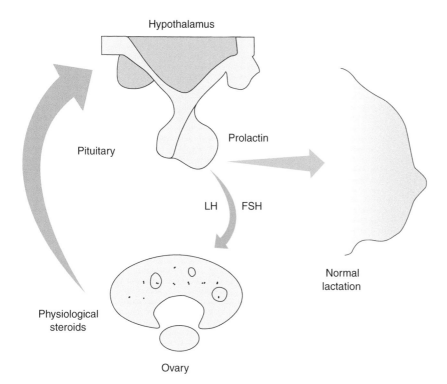

Figure 4.2   Hormonal cycles in the female

CONCEPTION, PREGNANCY, AND DELIVERY

All the eggs that a woman will release are set aside during fetal life. The male produces sperm from puberty to death. Sperm take approximately 120 days to mature. There are large variations in semen volume, sperm number, morphology, and motility. Apart from extreme values, the sperm count is not of great value as a predictor of fertility.

The many variations in female reproduction include differences in anatomy, physiology, and behavior. Human beings have a single uterine chamber, as opposed to the two horns found in many cattle (and in rare abnormalities in human beings); the cervix is firm and mucus-filled and ejaculation takes place in the vagina, whereas, in horses, the cervix admits the penis and ejaculation takes place in the uterus itself; the vagina is a single passage and not a double tube, as in kangaroos.

The human baby is immature, although not as blind and helpless as some other mammalian species (e.g. cats or bears). The human placenta is hemochorial, unlike say in pigs, where there is less erosion of the maternal and fetal tissues and less chance of severe hemorrhage during delivery as can so tragically affect human delivery.

THE MIRACLE OF LACTATION

'Mother', 'mummy', 'mamma', 'milk', all come from the same linguistic root: we belong to the zoological order Mammalia – and that means we breastfeed our babies.

The human infant depends for its life on its mother's milk. Milk not only nourishes the survival and growth of the child but also the fat content of the milk changes as the child matures and, for example, is adjusted to the needs of the growing brain. Milk is also loaded with antibodies (beginning with the colostrum) and maternal white cells that not only fight infection but also are tailored exactly to cure infections the mother has met in her environment. (The 'piglet in shit' survives because it receives protective antibodies from its mother living in the same unsanitary environment.) Milk also contains a factor that assists in the maturation of the baby's gut. Research shows that the protection given, if a mother breastfeeds for the first 3 months, against intestinal and respiratory infections persists until at least the end of the first year of life. Breastfeeding also reduces a mother's risk of breast cancer later in life.

It is the gonadotropin production from the early embryonic placenta which prevents the onset of the next menstruation; it is the pituitary hormones of the fetus which set the time of delivery. The newborn continues to be in control of the suckling process. The amount of suckling by the baby determines prolactin levels; this is the way by which the infant 'orders its next meal' and suckling is also the key factor in the suppression of ovulation during breastfeeding (Figure 4.3). As we have seen, in preliterate societies the duration of postpartum lactational amenorrhea is a key factor in the spacing of pregnancies, which in turn is a major factor in determining the risks of pregnancy to the mother and to

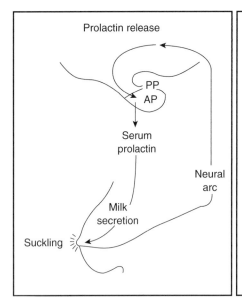
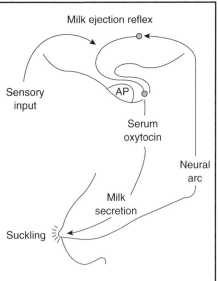

Prolactin release

Milk ejection reflex

Non-fertile state

Altered hypoyhalamic/pituitary function

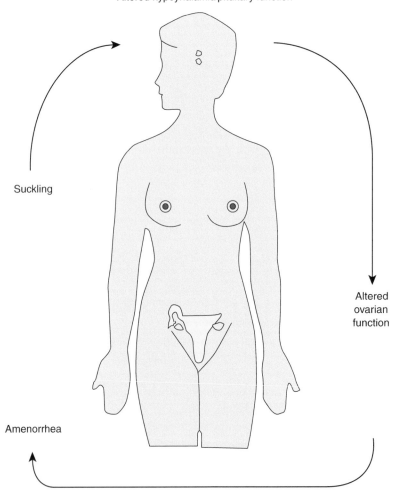

Suckling

Amenorrhea

Altered ovarian function

Figure 4.3 Diagrammatic representation of the pathways involved in suckling-induced prolactin and oxytocin release. Both hormones are released in response to nipple stimulation during suckling. The release of these hormones is otherwise independent. Prolactin release does not occur in response to other stimuli associated with nursing, while oxytocin release resulting in milk ejection may occur simultaneously or be induced by, for example, the cry of the infants. The non-fertile state diagram depicts how suckling alters the hypothalamic, pituitary and ovarian functions, in turn inducing lactational amenorrhea. From reference 1.

Table 4.1 Conditions for the lactational amenorrhea method (LAM)

The mother has not experienced vaginal bleeding after the 56th day post-partum
The baby is less than 6 months old
The baby receives all of its nutrition from the breast, without bottles, supplements, or solid food
The baby feeds at the breast at least every 4 hours during the day and every 6 hours at night

From reference 2, with permission.

the newborn infant, or the already existing older sibling. However, in order for lactation to be effective in preventing ovulation and a subsequent conception, there are specific criteria that must be met. These are explained in Table 4.1, and in further detail under the section on contraception in special groups, in Chapter 12.

Oral contraceptives mimic, albeit imperfectly, the natural suppression of ovulation occurring during pregnancy and breastfeeding. The fact that there is no similar interruption in the male production of sperm is the primary reason why we do not yet have a 'male pill'.

CHANGING PATTERNS OF REPRODUCTION

The time from the birth of one child until the birth of the next is called the birth interval (Figure 4.4). It consists of four parts:

1. The time taken to conceive.
2. The duration of pregnancy.
3. An interval without ovulation after delivery or abortion.
4. A possible period of secondary subfertility.

In the absence of contraception, most women fall pregnant within 3 months of beginning regular intercourse. In a traditional society not using contraceptives but breastfeeding for natural intervals, children are born 3–5 years apart. If breastfeeding is curtailed but not replaced by contraceptives, as in the North American Hutterites (a Protestant religious sect) then the average woman may have nine or ten live births in a lifetime.

An induced abortion prevents a birth but if the couple do not use contraceptives the woman may conceive again very rapidly and several abortions can occur in the same interval of time that it takes for a woman to conceive, deliver, and

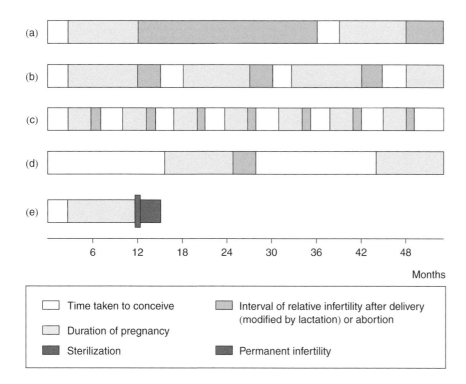

Figure 4.4 Patterns of human reproduction: (a) term delivery followed by breastfeeding; (b) term delivery followed by artificial feeding, wet-nursing or stillbirth; (c) spontaneous or induced abortion; (d) use of contraceptives; (e) pregnancy followed by voluntary sterilization.

Table 4.2 Percentages of adolescents reported to have experienced premarital coitus (selected countries)

Country and Year	Percent reporting any premarital intercourse – all women 15–19 years old	Percent reporting any premarital intercourse – all women 20–24 years old	Median age at first sexual intercourse – all women 20–24 years old	Median age at marriage – all women 20–24 years old
Benin 2001	41	55	17.2	19.1
Ethiopia 2001	3	10	18.1	18.1
Gabon 2000	56	73	16.2	20.4
Ghana 1998	27	54	17.5	19.3
Kenya 1998	37	66	17.3	20.2
Mali 1995–96	24	27	15.9	16.3
Bolivia 1998	13	39	19.6	20.9
Colombia 2000	30	59	18.4	21.4
Haiti 2000	25	54	18.2	20.6
Nicaragua 2001	9	22	18.1	18.7
Cambodia 2000	1	5	21.9	NA
Philippines 1998	2	9	22.8	NA

From references 3.

breastfeed a baby. Where abortion is combined with contraceptive use, the average time from initiating use until contraceptive failure becomes the largest element of the four components separating two pregnancies and the intervals represented by conception and abortion and conception and delivery are more nearly equivalent.

The increasing incidence of secondary subfertility, although unintended, also increases birth spacing. With reduced family size, widespread premarital sexual intercourse (Table 4.2), and late marriage, life-long patterns of reproduction in the West are now profoundly different from those characterizing earlier ages.

REFERENCES

1. http://www.fhi.org/training/en/modules/LAM/intro.htm
2. Better Breastfeeding, Healthier Lives. How programs and providers can help women improve breastfeeding practices. Population reports Series L, Number 14. Issues in World Health March 2006.
3. Population Reports, Volume XXXI, Number 2, Spring 2003 Series M, Number 17 Special Topics.

CHAPTER 5

Service delivery

Family planning involves three dynamic and interactive elements: fertility regulation methods, the nature of the service delivery system, and the perceptions and characteristics of the user (Figure 5.1). Experience shows that a change in a delivery system can be every bit as important in extending family planning choices as the invention of a new method. A new channel of distribution may meet the users' perceptions more closely, as when oral contraceptives are made available to men to give to their wives in a male-dominated society (Figure 5.2) or simply make it more convenient for users to obtain a method (Figure 5.3). The closest and quickest place to obtain contraceptives is often the neighborhood pharmacy or local store, where approximately 50% of the world's couples obtain their temporary family planning supplies (e.g. oral contraceptives, condoms, etc.). In both rich and poor countries most people have neither the time nor the inclination to travel long distances to obtain health care, let alone family planning services (Figure 5.4).

Health personnel have become unusually closely involved in family planning for two reasons: one licit and one accidental. Several methods (e.g. intrauterine devices or vasectomy) necessarily involve medical skills for their safe use. The accidental relationship is more subtle and probably also more important. When family planning is introduced into any community, it is commonly perceived as controversial and even socially disruptive (Chapter 3). Doctors, in particular, give family planning an air of respectability. Provider attitudes and availability of different contraceptive methods are linked closely and often remain more important than user perspectives in determining contraceptive availability and use in many countries. For example, it took the Japanese drug regulation authority 6 months to approve Viagra for sale, after it had systematically blocked the sale of oral contraceptives for 40 years. By the time the Pill was finally approved as a contraceptive, it had gathered a highly negative image and use is low even today (Figure 5.5).

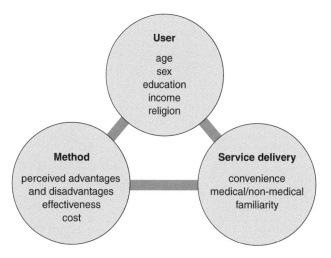

Figure 5.1 Family planning: an interaction between users, methods, and channels of delivery.

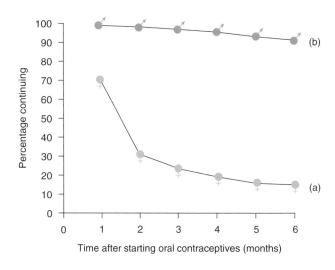

Figure 5.2 Continuation rate for oral contraceptive use in Iran: (a) oral contraceptives given by health personnel to women; (b) oral contraceptives given to husbands to pass to their wives.

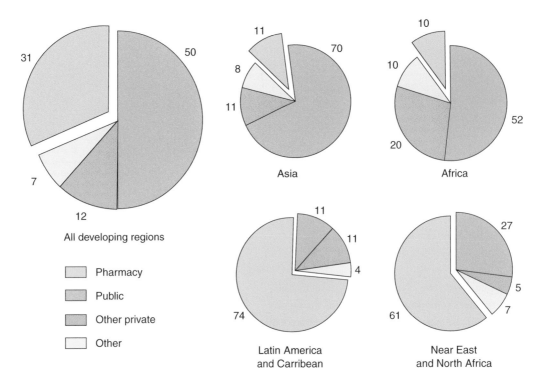

Figure 5.3 Users of condoms, oral contraceptives, injectables, or vaginal methods by source of supply (percentages) – estimates for developing areas. (From reference 1.)

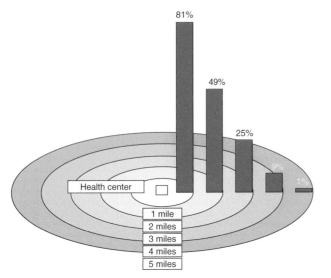

Figure 5.4 Utilization of health services (expressed as a percentage of health center clients) according to the distance traveled by the client.

Medical care, for good reason, is conservative and is necessarily overwhelmed by a diagnostic/therapeutic relationship between the physician and patient. Family planning is profoundly different and health professionals are no more than a 'fertility taxi driver' taking the user to their chosen fertility destination (Table 5.1).

To further complicate a confusing situation, physicians (e.g. Fernado Tamayo in Colombia, Sir Dougal Baird in the UK, Alan Guttmacher in the USA, and Jamo Yang in Korea)

Table 5.1 Paradigms in disease and family planning

Curative medicare	Family planning
Patient	User
Sickness	Health
Diagnosis by a health professional	Decision by user
Prescription of a therapy	Informed choice of method

Table 5.2 Barriers to access to contraception

Inappropriate eligibility criteria, including age and parity
Unwarranted contraindications
Unnecessary process hurdles including lab tests
Provider bias
Restrictions on providers
Regulatory barriers

have often been leaders in family planning, motivated by their personal, face-to-face experience of the anguish of unintended pregnancy and the pain of dangerous, exploitive abortions. But, at the same time, medical barriers to access to contraception (Table 5.2) have evolved into what may be the single most important impediment to the progress of family planning in many parts of the world.

It is easy to forget that in the middle of the last century specialized family planning clinics arose in Europe and North America because family planning was not an acceptable part of medical care. Today, the need is not to integrate other aspects of health care, such as STD (sexually transmitted

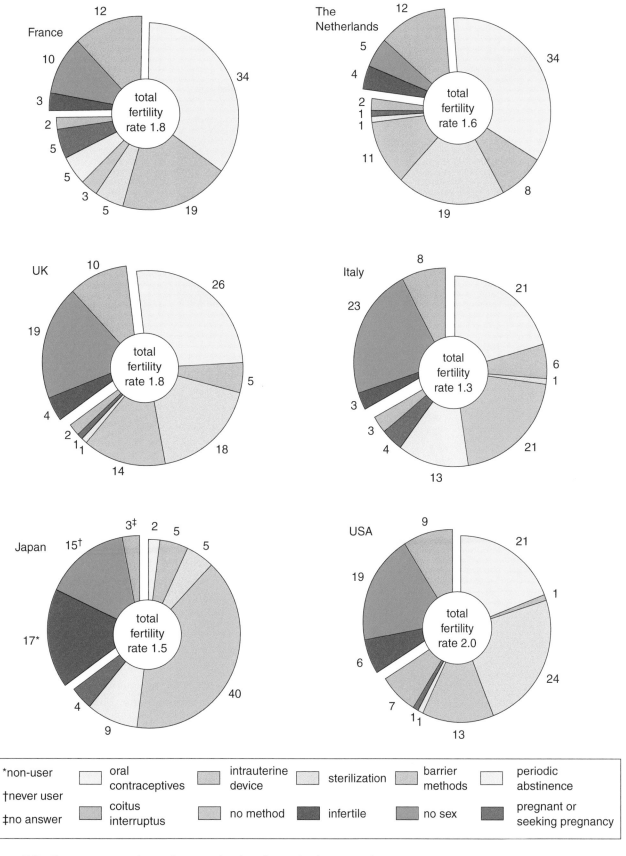

Figure 5.5 Current contraceptive use in women in selected countries (percentages).

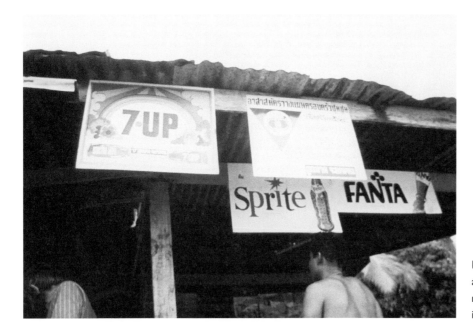

Figure 5.6 Condoms and pills are available in kiosks as part of the social marketing of the contraceptive program in Thailand.

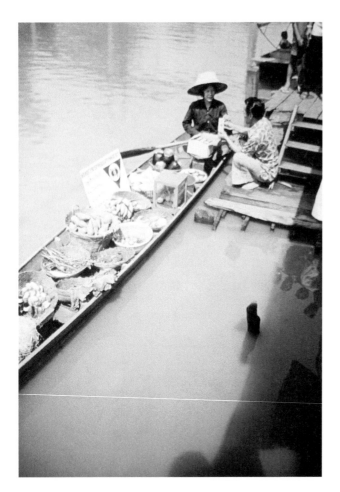

Figure 5.7 This lady travels the extensive Thai canal ways stopping at homes by the canal to sell her wares, including contraceptives, providing 'door-to-door' sales.

disease) control into family planning clinics, but to integrate family planning into mainstream medicine. Those countries where family planning has become part of the family medicine (e.g. the Netherlands) tend to have the highest use of contraception and the lowest induced abortion rates.

In practice, family planning benefits from the maximum diversity of channels of contraceptive distribution, and almost invariably the consumer will prove better at 'integrating' a variety of contraceptive services than any planner. Not only do people differ in their individual needs but also the same person, or couple, may get their fertility regulation from different sources as they make their life-long fertility journey: a young man may buy condoms from a slot machine, his fiancée may visit a family planning clinic for the pill, but get an intrauterine device from her gynecologist after their first child; she may choose an implant after their last wanted child, or her husband may go to a local clinic for a vasectomy.

Contraceptive advertising is sometimes forbidden by statute law, or industry guidelines. Some developing countries with national family planning programs still impose import duties on contraceptives.

In developing countries, social marketing (Figures 5.6 to 5.8) has brought condoms and pills into corner shops and kiosks, a community-based distribution service may serve vulnerable groups such as teenagers, and private doctors may provide abortions, and the government hospital voluntary surgical contraception. When the international community has helped subsidize family planning in resource-poor settings, typically it has given money to the Ministry of

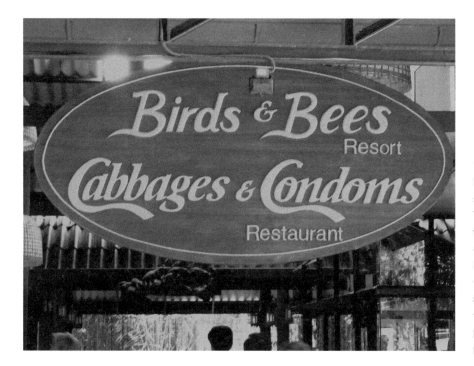

Figure 5.8 Under the imaginative leadership of Senator Mechai Viravaidya, sometimes called 'The condom king of Thailand', contraceptives have been transformed from embarrassing, under-the-counter items to open and acceptable items of everyday life. Cabbages and Condoms consists of two luxury hotels and a chain of restaurants in Thailand – the profits go toward subsidising family planning and rural development in the poor areas of the country.

Health or non-governmental organizations. However, some of the most successful family planning services, as in South Korea and Taiwan in the 1960s and 1970s adopted an output-based pattern of subsidy, where clients purchased a coupon or voucher at a low cost and then cashed it in a public clinic or private doctor of their choice. The provider sent the coupon to an agency that reimbursed them a realistic cost, for example to cover the real cost of IUD insertion. Output-based assistance is being explored once more, this time in Africa by the German Credit Bank and promises to be cost-effective, to enhance consumer choice (which helps improve the overall quality of services), and empowers the provider who can make their own decisions about the best way to use the money they earn.

Diversity is the key to access in family planning and pragmatism is the recurrent song of those seeking the maximum impact for their services. Wherever and however the service is provided, respect for the client is paramount. Every client should have a right to information, to access, to choice of method, to safety, to privacy, to confidentiality, to dignity, to comfort, to continuing services, and a right to express their opinion.

CHAPTER 6

Hormonal contraception

'THE PILL'

The principle of oral contraception was clearly described in the 1920s by Ludwig Haberlandt in Austria, but oral contraceptives came to fruition only in the 1950s with the availability of cheap sources of orally effective ovarian hormones. Even then, it took the drive of Margaret Sanger and the generosity of Paige McCormack of International Harvesters to persuade scientists at the Worcester Foundation in Boston, Massachusetts, to conduct the necessary research; and the obstetrician John Rock, the reproductive physiologist Gregory Pincus, and the scientist MC Chang to form a brilliant triumvirate which eventually provided women with a new and profoundly important contraceptive choice. Yet, when the initial clinical trials were conducted in Massachusetts, contraceptives were still illegal under the old Comstock laws; for this reason, research was transferred to Puerto Rico.

The early high-dose oral contraceptives were associated with rare but serious side effects, which often made media headlines and a realistic appraisal of the strengths and weaknesses of clinical trials and epidemiological studies of contraceptive effectiveness and safety remains important. Animal studies are difficult to interpret because of important differences in the reproductive systems of different species. The type of human trials conducted prior to drug registration by the UK Committee on Safety of Medicines or the US Food and Drug Administration (FDA) provide a good measure of failure rates and insight into short-term side effects – in the case of the pill, such things as nausea in the first few cycles of use and menstrual changes. Such trials, however, cannot detect rare events which might occur in one in 10 000 or even one in 1000 users. The introduction of new drugs and devices must be approached humbly and with caution and with an awareness that safety cannot be proved prior to widespread use.

We know now, that when used correctly and consistently, oral contraceptives are among the most effective reversible methods of contraception. However, reported pregnancy rates during the first year of use are as high as 32%. Because a major contributing factor to these oral contraceptive 'failures' is thought to be missed pills, researchers are attempting to determine how women's daily routines, interpretation of pill taking, or knowledge about oral contraceptives affects their pill use. Such information is needed so that family planning programs can help clients take oral contraceptives more consistently.

The main forms of oral contraception currently available include the combined oral contraceptives containing both estrogen and progestogen, the progestogen-only pill, and the hormonal postcoital pill for emergency use when a woman has been exposed to the risk of pregnancy.

Four decades after the introduction of the pill, more women than ever are using it. Currently more than 100 million women rely on the pill. It is the top modern family planning method among married women in half of countries surveyed.

Pill use in different countries of the world varies a great deal and estimates may not reveal the true picture. Rates of usage can vary from 2% in Japan to 34% in the Netherlands. The factors which determine pill use include biological factors such as family size and age; religion; medical, legal, and political aspects of the family planning program in the country; the availability and number of outlets where the pill can be obtained; and the amount of information – and misinformation – generated by the media.

Side effects – good and bad

In the case of oral contraceptives (OCs), epidemiological studies in the UK in the second half of the 1960s showed that these drugs had an adverse effect on the cardiovascular system. Deep vein thrombosis in the legs, heart attacks, and strokes were all slightly more common in users of high-dose oral contraceptives.

Modern oral contraceptives are safe for the great majority of women. The health risks of using OCs are much less than

Table 6.1   Factors to consider in starting or switching oral contraceptive pills

Objective	Action	Examples of products that achieve the objective
To minimize high risk of thrombosis	Select a product with a lower dosage of estrogen	Alesse, Loestrin 1/20, Levlite, Mircette
To minimize nausea, breast tenderness or vascular headaches	Select a product with a lower dosage of estrogen	Alesse, Levlite, Loestrin 1/20, Mircette
To minimize spotting or breakthrough bleeding	Select a product with a higher dosage of estrogen or a progestin with greater potency	Demulen, Desogen, Levlen, Lo/Ovral, Nordette, Ortho-Cept, Ortho-Cyclen, Ortho Tri-Cyclen
To minimize androgenic effects	Select a product containing a third-generation progestin, low-dose norethindrone, or ethynodiol diacetate	Brevicon, Demulen 1/35, Desogen,* Modicon, Ortho-Cept,* Ortho-Cyclen,* Ortho Tri-Cyclen,* Ovcon 35
To avoid dyslipidemia	Select a product containing a third-generation progestin, low-dose norethindrone or ethynodiol diacetate	Brevicon, Demulen 1/35, Desogen,* Modicon, Ortho-Cept,* Ortho-Cyclen,* Ortho Tri-Cyclen,* Ovcon 35

*These products contain a third-generation progestin.

*American Family Physician, November 1, 1999. Adapted From Hztcher et al.[2]

the risks of pregnancy and child-bearing for almost all women, especially in countries with high maternal mortality rates. Even where maternal mortality is low, pill use is safer than child-bearing except for older women who smoke or have high blood pressure. Today, with the lower doses in modern pills, the risks of a number of medical conditions appear to be lower than in the past. Also, recent large studies have made it possible to assess the health risks of long-term OC use more accurately and to better identify the groups most likely to experience them. A major finding of the last decade is the increased risk of heart attack and stroke for older OC users with hypertension. For OC users who do not smoke and do not have high blood pressure, however, the low doses in today's pills appear to minimize these risks.

The major established health risks of OCs are certain circulatory system diseases, particularly heart attack, stroke, and venous thromboembolism. Other health risks include gallbladder disease in women already susceptible to it and rare non-cancerous liver tumors. In addition, users and providers of OCs should be aware of possible interactions between OCs and other drugs that might make OCs less effective or modify the effects of the other drugs.[1]

The World Health Organization has developed a risk classification system to help physicians advise patients about the safety of oral contraceptive pills. The choice of pill formulation is influenced by clinical considerations. By choosing appropriately from the available pill formulations, family physicians can minimize negative side effects and maximize non-contraceptive benefits for their patients. Additional monitoring and follow-up are necessary in special populations, such as women over 35 years old, smokers, perimenopausal women, and adolescents. Third-generation progestins are additional options for achieving non-contraceptive benefits, but their use has raised new questions about thrombogenesis (Table 6.1).

The risk to the woman, while genuine, was comparable with or lower than that associated with the pregnancies that would inevitably occur if a woman used a less-effective method of contraception. In fact, risks associated with pill use are far lower than the risks taken almost daily when going about normal activities. Indeed, even things like using a ladder are far more dangerous than taking the modern low-dose OC; in the UK in 2002 approximately 35 000 people sought medical care for falling off a ladder and approximately 50 died[3] (Figure 6.1). The only exception was among women who smoked; smoking and oral contraceptive use have a marked adverse interaction, particularly in women over the age of 35 years. Once these effects were understood, the dose of hormones was rapidly and successfully reduced and screening methods, particularly in relation to age and smoking, eliminated most of the risks. In large-scale studies conducted in the late 1980s of newer low-dose pills correctly used, there was little or no evidence of any adverse cardiovascular effect. Nevertheless, previous experience has left both women and physicians with a markedly pessimistic view of oral contraceptives. Studies from around the world show that the majority of women think that taking the pill is more dangerous than having a pregnancy (Figure 6.2) and very few are aware of the non-contraceptive benefits of using the pill (Table 6.2).

The pill may well be the best-studied medication in history. After 40 years of use and with 100 million current users and an equal or greater number of women who have used the pill in the past, a vast and sometimes overwhelming amount of information exists, especially related to cancer and cardiovascular disease. It was always reasonable and necessary to explore the impact of oral contraceptives on reproductive cancers, although many unfounded and often frightening speculations were made in the past. Several factors influence the pattern of reproductive cancers, most

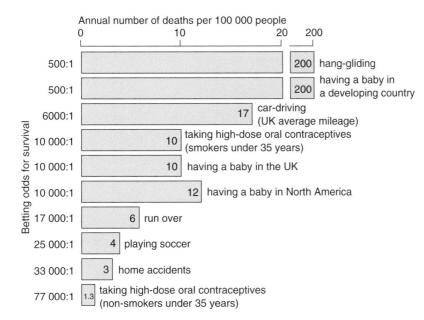

Annual number of deaths per 100 000 people

Betting odds for survival	value	label
500:1	200	hang-gliding
500:1	200	having a baby in a developing country
6000:1	17	car-driving (UK average mileage)
10 000:1	10	taking high-dose oral contraceptives (smokers under 35 years)
10 000:1	10	having a baby in the UK
10 000:1	12	having a baby in North America
17 000:1	6	run over
25 000:1	4	playing soccer
33 000:1	3	home accidents
77 000:1	1.3	taking high-dose oral contraceptives (non-smokers under 35 years)

Figure 6.1 Pill risks compared with other risks women run. These risks are lower, and possibly eliminated in the low-dose oral contraceptives now in widespread use. (From reference 1, with permission.)

Table 6.2 Non-contraceptive benefits of the combined oral contraceptive pill

The incidence of the following conditions is reduced	Potential benefits include protection against
Ovarian cancer	Osteoporosis
Endometrial cancer	Endometriosis
Pelvic inflammatory disease	Rheumatoid arthritis
Ectopic pregnancy	Toxic shock syndrome
Iron deficiency anemia	Fibroids
Benign breast disease	Colorectal cancer
Functional ovarian cyst	

unrelated to oral contraceptive use. The age of puberty, patterns of child-bearing, and age of menopause all have a marked effect on the incidence of breast, uterine, and ovarian cancer and it is reasonable and necessary to explore the possible effects of oral contraceptive use on these cancers. In the late 1980s, several studies consistently showed that use of the pill had a marked protective effect against ovarian and endometrial cancer.

OVARIAN & UTERINE CANCERS

The longer the pill is used, the greater is the reduction in the chance of developing ovarian and uterine cancer. The protection lasts for 10–15 years after taking the last pill and may even last for a lifetime. As these two cancers are also less frequent in women who have multiple pregnancies and long intervals of lactation, it seems that the pill, by suppressing ovulation, brings about the same pattern of protection.

Studies have consistently shown that using OCs reduces the risk of ovarian cancer. In a 1992 analysis of 20 studies of OC use and ovarian cancer, researchers from Harvard Medical School found that the risk of ovarian cancer decreased with increasing duration of OC use. Results showed a 10–12% decrease in risk after 1 year of use, and approximately a 50% decrease after 5 years of use.[5]

The use of OCs has been shown to significantly reduce the risk of endometrial cancer. This protective effect increases with the length of time OCs are used, and continues for many years after a woman stops using OCs.[6]

Combined OCs probably help protect against these cancers by reducing the rate of cell division in the endometrial lining and the ovaries. In the case of the uterine endometrium, the progestin component in the pill is thought to counteract the effects of estrogen, which would otherwise encourage cell division. OCs may protect against ovarian cancer by reducing gonadotropin production by the pituitary gland, thus reducing the effects of gonadotropin stimulation of the surface cells of the ovaries.

BREAST CANCER

A woman's risk of developing breast cancer depends on several factors, some of which are related to her natural hormones. Hormonal factors that increase the risk of breast cancer include conditions that may allow high levels of hormones to persist for long periods of time, such as beginning menstruation at an early age (before age 12),

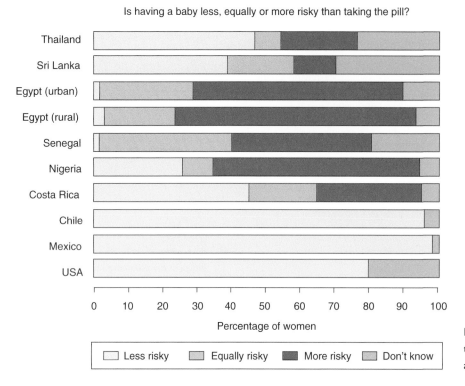

Is having a baby less, equally or more risky than taking the pill?

Percentage of women

Less risky   Equally risky   More risky   Don't know

Figure 6.2 The majority of women think taking the pill is more dangerous than having a pregnancy. (From reference 4.)

experiencing menopause at a late age (after age 55), having a first child after age 30, and not having children at all.

A 1996 analysis of worldwide epidemiological data conducted by the Collaborative Group on Hormonal Factors in Breast Cancer[7] found that women who were current or recent users of birth control pills had a slightly elevated risk of developing breast cancer. The risk was highest for women who started using OCs as teenagers. However, 10 or more years after women stopped using OCs, their risk of developing breast cancer returned to the same level as if they had never used birth control pills, regardless of family history of breast cancer, reproductive history, geographic area of residence, ethnic background, differences in study design, dose and type of hormone, or duration of use. In addition, breast cancers diagnosed in women after 10 or more years of not using OCs were less advanced than breast cancers diagnosed in women who had never used OCs.

The commonest reproductive cancer is that of the breast. According to the World Health Organization (WHO), more than 1.2 million people will be diagnosed with breast cancer this year worldwide. The American Cancer Society estimates that about 213 000 women in the USA will be diagnosed with invasive breast cancer each year (stages I–IV). The chance of developing invasive breast cancer during a woman's lifetime is approximately 1 in 8 (about 13%). Another 62 000 women will be diagnosed with in-situ breast cancer, a very early form of the disease.[8] Death rates for lung cancer and breast cancer are given in Figure 6.3.

Cancer of the breast became more common in every decade in the 20th century and the vast majority of women who have suffered this scourge of death and illness have been too old ever to have taken oral contraceptives. When all the women who have used the pill are compared with non-users, then no adverse or beneficial effect of the pill in relation to breast cancer has been demonstrated (Figure 6.4). In the small group of women who are unfortunate enough to develop breast cancer before the age of 35 years, and who also used the pill early in their reproductive life, some studies show a slight increase in risk while others show no effect. It is also possible that the first pregnancy is associated with a slight short-term rise in the risk of breast cancer, followed by a longer-term statistically more significant protective effect.

CERVICAL CANCER

Many, perhaps most, cervical cancers are caused by viral infections, and cervical cancer rates are related to the number of sexual partners, or to the number of sexual partners of the woman's husband/partner. Some studies have found a higher rate of cervical cancer in oral contraceptive users; however, this may reflect a higher number of sexual partners in oral contraceptive users rather than a direct causal effect.

Evidence shows that long-term use of OCs (≥ 5 years) may be associated with an increased risk of cancer of the cervix (the narrow, lower portion of the uterus). Although

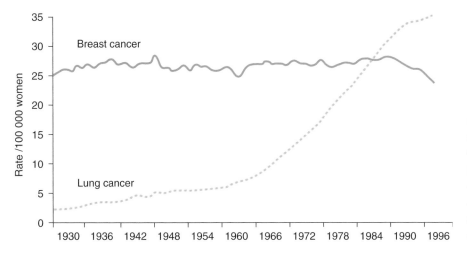

Figure 6.3 Age-adjusted death rates for lung cancer and breast cancer among women in the USA, 1930–1997.
Note: Death rates are age-adjusted to the 1970 population. Sources: Parker et al, 1996; National Center for Health Statistics, 1999; Riess et al, 2000; American Cancer Society, unpublished data

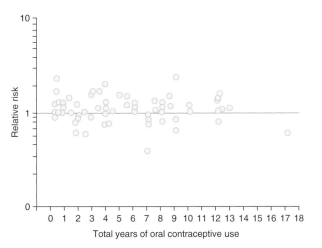

Figure 6.4 Breast cancer in women younger than 60 years of age: relative risk by total years of oral contraceptive use in 17 studies since 1980.

OC use may increase the risk of cervical cancer, human papillomavirus (HPV) is recognized as the major cause of this disease. Approximately 14 types of HPV have been identified as having the potential to cause cancer, and HPVs have been found in 99% of cervical cancer biopsy specimens worldwide. More information about HPV and cancer is available in Human Papillomaviruses and Cancer: Questions and Answers.[9,10]

A 2003 analysis by the International Agency for Research on Cancer (IARC) found an increased risk of cervical cancer with longer use of OCs. Researchers analyzed data from 28 studies that included 12 531 women with cervical cancer. The data suggested that the risk of cervical cancer may decrease after OC use stops.[11] In another IARC report, data from eight studies were combined to assess the effect of OC use on cervical cancer risk in HPV-positive women. Researchers found a fourfold increase in risk among women who had used OCs for longer than 5 years. Risk was also increased among women who began using OCs before age 20 and women who had used OCs within the past 5 years.[12] The IARC is planning a study to reanalyze all data related to OC use and cervical cancer risk.[13]

LIVER CANCER

How do oral contraceptives affect liver cancer risk?

Several studies have found that OCs increase the risk of liver cancer in populations usually considered low risk, such as white women in the USA and Europe who do not have liver disease. In these studies, women who used OCs for longer periods of time were found to be at increased risk for liver cancer. However, OCs did not increase the risk of liver cancer in Asian and African women, who are considered high risk for this disease. Researchers believe this is because other risk factors, such as hepatitis infection, outweigh the effect of OCs.[14]

WORLD WIDE USE

The picture which has emerged in the study of the pill and cancer is that oral contraceptive use, like pregnancy, changes the pattern of reproductive cancers, making ovarian and uterine cancer substantially less common and breast cancer slightly more common. An overall picture taking into account the cardiovascular risks, the changing pattern of reproductive cancers and the obvious protection against the risks of pregnancy and childbirth is difficult to establish, but, on average, a woman who uses the pill for some years may reduce her expectation of life by at most a few tens of days. For comparison, an individual who smokes a pack of cigarettes a day reduces their average expectation of life by over

4 years. Another way of looking at pill risk is to point out that even the old high-dose pills carried less risk than smoking one cigarette a day.

In many countries, the pill can now be obtained as an over-the-counter item, like the condom. In the West commercial manufacturers prefer to distribute oral contraceptives as prescription products which are more profitable, but there are no scientific reasons why oral contraceptives should not be sold over-the-counter beside the extra-strength Tylenol and similar easy to obtain medications. The fact that older women who smoke should use an alternative method of contraception can be written on the package, and sooner or later developed countries are likely to switch oral contraceptives from their current prescription status to over-the-counter sale. The adage that the pill should be in slot machines and cigarettes on prescription remains a sound one.

COMBINED ORAL CONTRACEPTIVES

The most widely used oral preparations are those containing estrogen and progestogen taken in constant amounts for 20, 21, or 22 days followed by an interval without steroids during which uterine bleeding occurs. The commonest regimen is a 21-day course, followed by an interval of 7 days when no tablet is taken, or placebo, iron and/or vitamin tablets are substituted. The tendency in recent years has been to reduce the dose of both estrogen and progestogen, with some currently available preparations having the minimum effective dose.

Phasic preparations, with a changing dose of progestogen, allow the use of smaller amounts of steroids while still maintaining good cycle control. These pills attempt to mimic the normal cycle and have an initial estrogen dominance. They require slightly more compliance in use.

Today's low-dose combined oral contraceptives contain less than 50 μg estrogen, down from 150 μg in the first oral contraceptive and 50–100 μg in those of the late 1960s and the 1970s.

Estrogen doses of 30–35 μg ethinylestradiol are the most common. Some low-dose pills use 50 μg mestranol, which is roughly as potent as 35 μg ethinylestradiol. Progestin doses have also dropped substantially. For example, doses of norethindrone have dropped from 10 mg to 1.0 or 0.5 mg. Because progestins vary in potency by weight, doses of other progestins range from 0.05 to 2.0 mg.

Low-estrogen oral contraceptives are now the most widely used. Data from 37 countries in 1987 suggest that low-estrogen pills accounted for nearly 85% of pharmacy sales of oral contraceptives in the developed countries and almost 60% in the developing countries. In 1988 they constituted almost 80% of oral contraceptives donated to family planning programs in developing countries.

MODE OF ACTION

The primary action of combined oral contraceptive pills is the cessation of ovulation brought about by the inhibition of pituitary follicle-stimulating hormone (FSH), thus inhibiting follicular maturation in the ovary, and by the abolition of the estrogen-mediated positive feedback, which is the physiological trigger for the ovulatory surge of luteinizing hormone (LH) (Figures 6.5 and 6.6). Seven consecutive pills are sufficient to inhibit ovulation. Cervical mucus is also affected, mainly by the progestogen component, and rendered

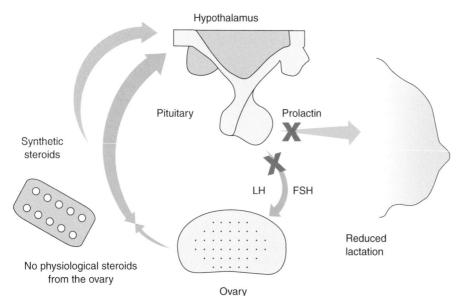

Figure 6.5 Alteration of hormonal cycles by oral contraception.

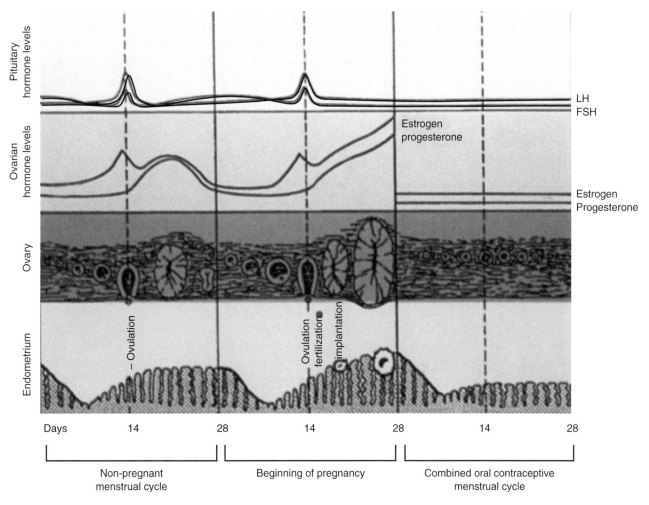

Figure 6.6 A diagrammatic comparison showing changes which occur in the endometrium, ovary, and in plasma hormone levels during the non-pregnant menstrual cycle, the beginning of pregnancy, and the oral contraceptive menstrual cycle. LH, luteinizing hormone; FSH, follicle stimulating hormone. (From reference 15, with permission.)

inhospitable to sperm. The receptivity of the endometrium to the blastocyst is also reduced. These latter two mechanisms act as a back-up to the main ovarian effect.

Advantages and disadvantages

When choosing a method of contraception, a potential user must have access to up-to-date objective information on advantages and disadvantages. The pill has a number of short-term advantages and disadvantages which users should understand (Tables 6.3 and 6.4). The longer-term non-contraceptive benefits of the combined oral contraceptive pill are outlined in Table 6.2. Women using the pill have a flattened endometrium and, therefore, the periods are both regular and reduced in volume compared with in women who do not use hormonal contraceptives. It has been known for 40 years and clinically demonstrated for 30, that once a woman starts using the pill it is safe and

Table 6.3 Short-term advantages of the combined oral contraceptive pill

Acne is improved with some pills
Breast tenderness is usually reduced
100% protection against pregnancy is assured
Intercourse is unaffected
Regular menstruation
Timing of menstruation can be controlled
No ovulation pain
Less premenstrual tension
Less period pain
Less heavy bleeding, therefore less anemia
Less pelvic infection
100% reversible
Can be used for treatment of dysfunctional uterine bleeding

responsible to choose any pattern of menstruation she wishes. By omitting placebo (or iron tablets) and continuing to take active tablets uterine bleeding can be postponed for

Table 6.4 Short-term disadvantages of the combined oral contraceptive pill

Amenorrhea
Midcycle spotting
Depression
Fluid retention/bloatedness
Headaches
Reduced libido in some users
Migraine
Nausea in the first month of use
Weight gain

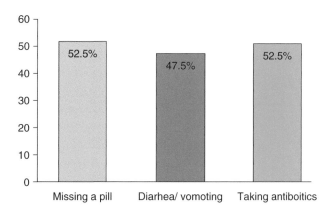

Figure 6.7 Percentage of users of the pill who are unaware of the consequences of missing a pill, if antibiotics are being taken, or if diarrhea and/or vomiting is occurring. (From reference 4, with permission.)

months or years. One branded product is packaged to give four periods a year.

Over the years and partly propelled by medicolegal considerations, the FDA and other national drug regulatory authorities have required manufacturers to provide useful information about benefits of oral contraceptive use. Side effects and contraindications to pill use are outlined in Tables 6.4 and 6.5.

The pill is only effective if taken correctly and consistently. Many studies have shown, however, that many users are not fully aware of what they should do if they forget to take a pill or delay taking it, and also what should be done if the user has diarrhea or vomits the pill (Figure 6.8). If users forget to take the pill, then loss of efficacy may be pronounced for the next 7 days or more if pills are omitted early in a packet (Table 6.6).

CONTINUOUS-USE ORAL CONTRACEPTIVES

More and more reproductive health experts are questioning the necessity for the monthly withdrawal bleed, which OC users experience while taking the seven inactive

Table 6.5 Contraindications of combined oral contraception

Absolute contraindications	*Relative contraindications*
Abnormal vaginal bleeding of unknown etiology	Diabetes mellitus
Cerebrovascular disease	Epilepsy
Congenital hyperlipidemia	Gall bladder disease
Coronary occlusion	Morbid obesity
Estrogen-responsive tumors (breast, ovarian, uterine, etc.)	Obstructive jaundice in prior pregnancy
Hepatic neoplasms	Severe hypertension up to 180 mmHg
Impaired liver function	Severe vascular headache
Smoker older than 35 years	
Thrombophlebitis/ thromboembolic disease	

From reference 16.

pills or 7 days without pills in each month's cycle. New research has found that women can safely and effectively use many monophasic OCs continuously for a few cycles in a row, skipping the inactive pills. ('Monophasic' means that each active pill in the cycle contains the same amount of hormones.)

The monthly regimen of 21 active pills containing estrogen and progestin, followed by seven inactive pills, was created to promote monthly withdrawal bleeding and to mimic spontaneous menstrual cycles. Taking active pills continuously allows women to reduce the number of times they experience monthly bleeding per year and to reduce the number of bleeding days. Continuous-use OCs also significantly reduce the side effects associated with hormone withdrawal, including migraines, headaches, premenstrual syndrome, mood changes, and heavy or painful monthly bleeding, which women experience primarily on the days they take the inactive pills.

Women taking OCs continuously are about twice as likely as women using the conventional regimen to have breakthrough bleeding between periods, which leads many to discontinue use. Breakthrough bleeding and spotting diminish after about 8 or 9 months of use; however, researchers have studied a few different OCs for continuous use with different results in controlling breakthrough bleeding and other side effects.

One formulation, Seasonique, is packaged specifically for continuous use and is FDA approved (Figure 6.8). It contains 150 μg of the progestin levonorgestrel and 30 μg of the estrogen ethinyl estradiol. Seasonique users take a pill every day for 84 days (12 weeks) and then take hormone-free pills for 7 days. Only 10 months after Seasonique became available, more than 260 000 prescriptions for it had been written in the US. Its developer,

Table 6.6 What to do in case of a missed pill (combined oral contraceptive containing 30–35 mg ethinylestradiol).

Missed one or two pills
She should take a pill as soon as possible and then continue taking pills daily, one each day*
She does not need any additional contraceptive protection

Missed three or more pills
She should take a pill as soon as possible and then continue taking pills daily, one each day[†]
She should also use condoms or abstain from sex until she has taken pills for 7 days in a row
If she missed the pills in the third week, she should finish the pills in her current pack and start a new pack the next day. She should
    not have a pill-free interval. If the pill-free interval is avoided in this way, she does not need to use emergency contraception
If she missed the pills in the first week (effectively extending the pill-free interval) and had unprotected sex (in week 1 or in the
    pill-free interval), she may wish to consider the use of emergency contraception

For everyday pill regimens
If a woman misses any inactive pills, she should discard the missed inactive pills and then continue taking pills daily, one each day

*If a woman misses more than one pill, she can take the first missed pill and then either continue taking the rest of the missed pills or discard them to stay on schedule.
[†]Depending on when she remembers that she missed a pill(s), she may take two pills on the same day (one at the moment of remembering, and the other at the regular time, or even at the same time).

Barr Laboratories, plans to apply for approval in other countries.[19]

PROGESTOGEN-ONLY PILLS

The progestogen-only pills are estrogen-free oral contraceptives containing a microdose of progestogen from either the norethindrone or levonorgestrel group. The first progestogen-only pill was introduced in 1969. The progestogen-only pill has to be taken daily and at a regular time without a 7-day break. It may make it easier for women to adhere to a regular pill-taking pattern.

The efficacy of the progestogen-only pill is less than that of the combined oral contraceptive. Failure rates vary between 0.3 and 5.0 per 100 woman-years. They exert their main action on the cervical mucus, leading to the production of thick mucus with poor sperm penetrability. Ovulation may also be inhibited in approximately 60% of women.

The main side effect of the progestogen-only pill is an irregular bleeding cycle, and in some women amenorrhea can result.

Progestogen-only pills combine good efficiency with lack of major side effects and minimal alteration in metabolic effects. They may be particularly suitable for women who have side effects or contraindications to the combined oral contraceptives, in particular those side effects believed to be estrogen-related. Therefore, they can safely be used in smokers over 35 years of age, as well as in women who are at an increased risk of thromboembolism. Progestogen-only pills are suitable for older women, mainly over the age of 40 years, and for women during lactation.

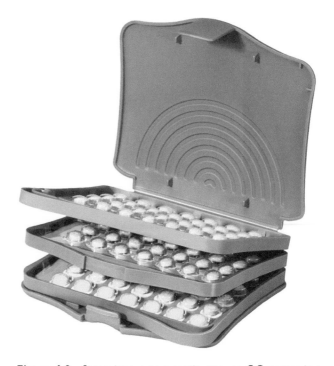

Figure 6.8 Seasonique, a new continuous-use OC, comes in a 3-month supply. Women take one active pill per day for 84 days and then take inactive pills for 7 days. Continuous-use OCs reduce the number of bleeding days and related side effects. (Courtery of Barr Laboratories.)

EMERGENCY (POSTCOITAL) CONTRACEPTION

Emergency (postcoital) contraception using orally administered hormones is considered to be a one-time procedure and not a routine approach to contraception. The widely used preparation on the market today contains 750 mg of levonorgestrel in each tablet. As compared with the previously marketed PC4 (ethinyl estradiol and progestogen containing preparation), this has relatively fewer cumbersome side-effects such as nausea and vomiting, which is no doubt the reason for its current popularity. Four tablets should be taken within 24 hours of intercourse. It is known that emergency contraception works better the sooner it is used, and the quickest way for some women, for whom access to pharmacies is difficult, is to use eight low-dose oral contraceptive tablets from their sister's or best friend's pack. (The donor of the tablets may either throw away the rest of the pack and start a new pack, or use the remaining tablets and then continue to a new pack omitting the placebo, inert tablets.) The failure rate, which is around 0.4% if treatment is complied with within 24 hours, increases by a further 50% with each 12-hour delay (Figure 6.9).[19,20]

The most recent WHO guidelines state that a single dose of levonorgestrel (1.5 mg) is the best regimen for emergency contraception, probably due to higher preference and compliance by clients, and fewer side effects such as vomiting.

Emergency contraception is suitable for women exposed to unprotected sexual intercourse. It is of particular value in preventing pregnancy and the consequent psychological distress in females who have been subjected to rape (see Contraception in situation of humanitarian crises in Chapter 12). The new WHO guidance supports previous advice to take the emergency contraceptive pill ideally within 72 hours, but recent research shows that it can be effective if taken up to 120 hours (5 days after the unprotected sexual exposure). Standard contraindications to the use of combined hormonal contraceptives should be observed. Possible side effects include nausea, vomiting, irregular uterine bleeding, breast tenderness, and headache.

Ideally, the woman should be seen a month later for counseling for elective contraception and to exclude the possibility of pregnancy.

LONG-ACTING HORMONAL METHODS

Injectables

Ovarian hormones are more easily delivered systemically than orally. A comparison of the effects of the combined pill, the progestogen-only pill, and injectable preparations is shown in Table 6.7, and the mechanism of action of injectables is shown in Figure 6.10. The problem with injectables is how to obtain a regular release over a long interval of time. The two most commonly used intramuscular injectable preparations are a 3-monthly injection of a relatively high dose of medroxyprogesterone acetate (MPA) (150 mg in a microcrystalline suspension; Depo-Provera,

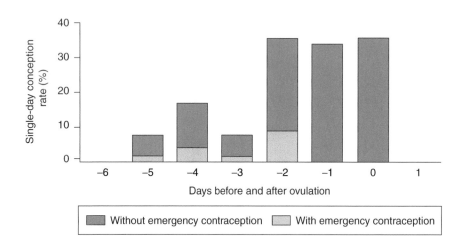

Figure 6.9 Probability of conception with the use of the emergency contraceptive pill. (From reference 18.)

Table 6.7 Comparison of action of contraceptive hormone preparations

Effects	Combined pill	Progestogen-only pill	Injectable
Ovulation suppressed	Yes	No	Yes
Endometrial changes	Yes	Yes	Yes
Cervical mucus changes	Yes	Yes	Yes
Lactation suppressed	Yes	No	No
Pregnancy rate per woman-years in use	0.5–5.0	2–10	1.0

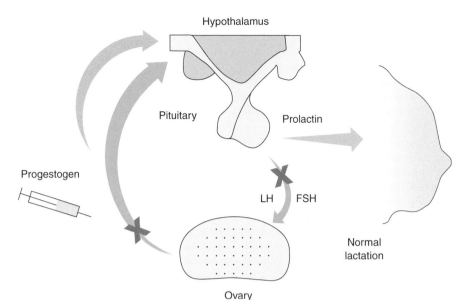

Figure 6.10 Alteration of hormonal cycles by injectables.

Megestron) and a 2-monthly injection of norethindrone enanthate (200 mg in oil; NET-OEN, Noristerat, Norigest).

Injectable contraceptive formulations

In 1991, the United Nations Population Fund estimated that injectable contraceptives were used by close to 13 million women in the developing world. They include approximately 10 million users of the 3-monthly preparation, depot-medroxyprogesterone acetate (DMPA), 2 million users of the NET-EN, and 1 million users of once-a-month injectable preparations.

Injectables: today and tomorrow

More and more women are using injectable contraceptives today, and very likely even more will use this method in the future as it becomes increasingly available. Women choose injectables because they are effective, long-lasting, and private. For family planning programs, meeting increasing demand while maintaining good quality will be the key to success with injectables.

Between 1995 and 2005 the number of women worldwide using injectable contraceptives more than doubled. About 12 million married women used injectables in 1995. In 2005 over 32 million were using injectables. Injectables are the fourth most popular method worldwide, after female sterilization, the intrauterine device (IUD), and oral contraceptives. In Sub-Saharan Africa, injectables are the most popular method chosen by 38% of women using modern methods. By 2015, worldwide use is projected to reach nearly 40 million – more than triple the 1995 level.

Greater access largely explains this rapid growth in use. Approval of the progestin-only injectable DMPA in the USA in 1992 removed a constraint to access and a source of controversy in many countries over providing a drug that was not approved for contraception in the USA. Also, approval in the USA enabled the US Agency for International Development (USAID) to supply DMPA to developing countries. As of 2006, DMPA was registered in 179 countries, an increase from 106 countries in 1995. Several countries, including Ghana, Vietnam, and Zambia, are introducing or scaling up DMPA services as part of a package of reproductive or primary health care services.

In the next 10 years more family planning programs will offer injectables, and they will offer clients more choices of injectables. Most can be expected to offer a progestin-only injectable – DMPA injected every 3 months or NET-EN injected every 2 months. Many will offer a combined injectable, probably either MPA combined with the estrogen estradiol cypionate (E_2C) or NET-EN combined with the estrogen estradiol valerate (E_2V). Both are injected monthly. Other combined injectables are available in some countries and regions (Table 6.8).

Progress was made to develop levonorgestrel butanoate as a new injectable hormonal contraceptive that will have a duration of action of up to 3 months after a single 10 mg dose. Such a low-dose preparation would expose a woman to a lesser amount of synthetic hormone than is the case with DMPA, the currently available 3-monthly injectable. The lower dose would also result in less suppression of the ovaries, which in turn would result in fewer women experiencing amenorrhea. In addition, fertility would be restored more rapidly after stopping the injections than is the case with DMPA.

Depo-Provera is off-patent and several generic manufacturers exist. It has an exceptionally low failure rate (under 1%) but it also takes some time to eliminate all the

Table 6.8 Formulations, injection schedules, and availability of injectable contraceptives

Common trade names	Formulation	Injection type and schedule	Registration/availability in 2006
Progestin-only injectables			
Depo-Provera, Megestron, Contracep, Depo-Prodasone	Depot medroxyprogesterone acetate (DMPA) 150 mg	One intramuscular (IM) injection every 3 months	Registered in 179 countries
Depo-subQ Provera 104 (DMPA-SC)	DMPA 104 mg	One subcutaneous injection every 3 months	Approved in the USA and the UK; approval expected soon in other European countries; expected to be available in some developing countries by 2008
Noristeral, Norigest, Doryxas	Norethisterone enanthate (NET-EN) 200 mg	One IM injection every 2 months	Registered in 91 countries
Combined injectables (progestin + estrogen)			
Cyclofem, Ciclofeminina, Lunelle	Medroxyprogesterone acetate 25 mg + estradiol cypionate 5 mg (MPA/E$_2$C)	One IM injection every month	Registered in 12 countries[b]
Mesigyna, Norigynon	NET-EN 50 mg + estradiol valerate 5 mg (NET-EN/E$_2$V)	One IM injection every month	Registered in 33 countries
Deladroxate, Perlutal, Topasel, Patectro, Deproxone, Nomagest	Dihydroxyprogesterone (algestone) acetophenide 150 mg + estradiol enanthate 10 mg	One IM injection every month	Registered in 14 Latin American countries and Spain
Anafertin, Yectames	Dihydroxyprogesterone (algestone) acetophenide 75 mg + estradiol enanthate 5 mg	One IM injection every month	Registered in 7 Latin American countries
Chinese Injectable No. 1	17α-hydroxyprogesterone caproate 250 mg + estradiol valerate 5 mg	One IM injection every month, except 2 injections in first month	Registered in China

From reference 21. Population Reports, December 2006, Expanding Services for Injectables.

hormone after the last injection and there is some delay in the return of fertility, although there is no evidence of any long-term impairment. Norethindrone enanthate uses a slightly lower dose of progestogen but is less tolerant of delays between injections, and the injection needs to be repeated after 2 rather than 3 months. Contraindications of long-acting preparations include hypertension, diabetes, and large fibroids; side effects include irregular bleeding, amenorrhea, delayed return of ovulation, hypertension, and changes in carbohydrate metabolism. As these preparations lack estrogens, they appear to have no adverse effect on the cardiovascular system. Like any contraceptives they should not be used if there is a suspicion of pregnancy.

Monthly injectables, which usually contain lower doses of a long-acting progestogen and a small dose of a shorter-acting estrogen, are now available since their FDA approval in 2000. They give rise to a more regular bleeding pattern. Examples of this type of formulation include:

1. Norethindrone enanthate 50 mg + estradiol valerate 5 mg.
2. Depot medroxyprogesterone acetate 25 mg + estradiol cypionate 4 mg.
3. Dihydroxyprogesterone acetophenide 150 mg + estradiol enanthate 10 mg.

The WHO has developed a monthly injectable, Cyclofem, combining an already known progestogen, depot medroxyprogesterone acetate 25 mg and a known estrogen, estradiol cypionate 5 mg. This has been available in Mexico, Thailand, and Indonesia since 1993 and is now being used in many other countries. In addition, a once-a-month injectable Mesigyna containing norethindrone enanthate 50 mg and estradiol valerate 5 mg is also now available. These are highly effective contraceptives which achieve better cycle control than the longer-acting injectables, and a more rapid return to ovulation once discontinued. However, monthly injectables have the disadvantage of requiring more frequent administration. In order to prevent spread of infection when giving injectable contraceptives, health workers are advised to use disposable syringes and needles. However, due to costs and shortage of syringes and needles, many developing countries continue to reuse equipment, and thus the spread of infection is known to take place. To eliminate the problem of reusing needles and syringes, a single-use prefilled syringe for long-term injectables has been developed (Figure 6.11).[22]

Once-a-month combined injectable preparations draw their contraceptive efficacy from continuous ovulation suppression. When their use is discontinued, ovulation resumes within a few weeks or a few months, depending on the formulation. After use of the dihydroxyprogesterone acetophenide 150 mg + estradiol enanthate 5 mg combination for 1–2 years, ovulation returns in most subjects 3–4 months after discontinuation of treatment. Similarly, recent data show that after 2-year use of the depot-medroxyprogesterone acetate 25 mg + estradiol cypionate 5 mg or the norethisterone enanthate 50 mg + estradiol valerate 5 mg combination, approximately 70% women have resumed ovulation by the third month post-treatment. This is shorter than the time for return of ovulation experienced by ex-users of progestogen-only injectable contraceptives.

Injectable use has been literally dogged by adverse headlines coming from studies on Depo-Provera given to beagle dogs, and as a result many women who would have benefited greatly from its use have been denied the choice. When the drug industry first started doing long-term cancer studies in animals in the 1950s and 1960s they chose beagle dogs for no better reason than the fact that they are good-natured and tolerate laboratory routines without biting the attendants! Physiologically they were a disastrous choice. They happen to be a species in which, even without any intervention, there is a high rate of spontaneous breast cancer. Unlike human beings, where reproduction is independent of the season, bitches are seasonal breeding animals and the sexual cycle is fairly different from that of primates. The occurrence of breast cancer in beagles given high doses of Depo-Provera confused scientists and alarmed the public. Sincere consumer groups argued that the method was dangerous and, in particular, should not be given to women in poor countries.

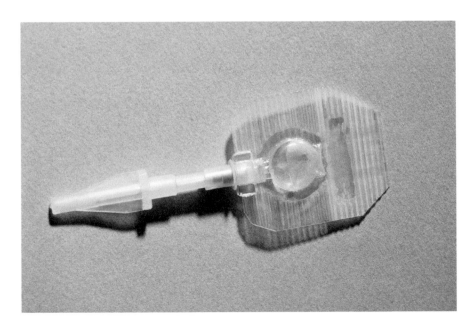

Figure 6.11 An example of a single-use prefilled syringe. It can be used for long-acting injectable contraceptives. (Courtesy of The Program for Applied Technology in Health.)

Beagle dogs are no longer required as test animals by any national drug regulatory authority. Injectable contraceptives have been licensed in the majority of the world's countries, from Chile to Britain to Thailand to New Zealand. Large-scale case–control studies of women with cancer in Third World countries have shown injectables behave like oral contraceptives. Like the pill, injectable contraceptives probably reduce the risk of ovarian and uterine cancer and, as they lack the estrogenic effects, they may, overall, be even safer. In 1992, the expert committee advising the FDA once again recommended approval of Depo-Provera as a contraceptive for women in the USA, and finally, 28 years after the first recommendation (1965), Depo-Provera became available to women in the USA as a contraceptive. Undoubtedly, a great many women have died from childbirth and abortion whose lives might have been saved had injectable contraceptives been fully understood at an early stage in their history.

Long-acting injectable contraceptives are highly effective. Serum iron levels are noted to be increased during use of these drugs. The advantages are listed in Table 6.9. The disadvantages, on the other hand, are relatively few. They cause a change in menstrual patterns, inducing amenorrhea or spotting. A potential disadvantage is the inability to withdraw the drug promptly. Long-term use may be associated with some increase in osteoporosis. There is also the potential for abuse by health practitioners who may not always tell the user all the disadvantages. Once the injection has been given, the woman has no control over the method, other than to wait until the effects wear off. Long-acting injectables are not practical for self-administration.

Implants

Subcutaneous implants with constant slow release of a variety of different progestogens have been shown to provide excellent contraception.

Contraceptive implants have been approved in more than 60 countries and are being used by approximately 11 million women worldwide.

The main advantage of implants over other methods of contraception is their extremely high degree and long duration of efficacy following insertion. In addition, the doses of progestogen they deliver are lower than those given in oral and injectable contraceptives and blood levels are very stable over long periods.

Among the drawbacks of implants is the need for a surgical procedure for their insertion and removal. Although the procedure is a minor one, it should only be performed by trained personnel and it can therefore be relatively costly.

The most notable drawback of implants, however, and the one that most women invoke as a reason for discontinuing

Table 6.9 Advantages of long-acting contraceptives

Post injection infertility lasting 4–9 months

No known interference with lactation

No increased risk of cancer

Protection against pelvic inflammatory disease

Protection against ovarian/endometrial cancer

No estrogen-related side-effects

Elimination of user error (i.e. user compliance is not a factor)

Use is not coitus-related

Infrequent administration – an advantage in prolonged use

High degree of privacy (no supplies need to be kept around the house)

A clinical setting is not required for provision of this method of contraception

Injectables are acceptable forms of medication in many cultures

Absorption of the drug is not dependent on normal gastrointestinal function

Pregnancy rates are low

No mortality has been associated with their use

the method, is the high prevalence (in 11–12% of users) of menstrual problems. These problems are typical of all contraceptives that use only progestogen, as distinct, say, from oral contraceptives that use a combination of a progestogen and an estrogen.

Menstrual problems range from amenorrhea to frequent, irregular, heavy, or prolonged bleeding. However, total blood loss is generally lower than from normal menstruation. A cluster of side effects, including headache, weight change, and acne, is the second most frequent reason for discontinuation.

These implants have usually consisted of silastic capsules packed with crystalline steroid. The 5-year levonorgestrel-releasing system (Norplant) developed by the Population Council has been available in many countries for some time (Figure 6.14). The recent WHO Progress in Reproductive health has mentioned that these implants can remain in place for up to 7 years in women who weigh less than 70 kg.

Since the advent of the six-rod containing Norplant, two other forms of hormonal implants have been manufactured and approved for use. The two-rod hormonal implant (Jadelle) acts for a period of 5 years, and the single rod Implanon can be used for 3 years (see below).

Jadelle, which, like Norplant, was also developed by Population Council researchers and is identical to Norplant except for having two rods instead of six capsules releasing levonorgestrel. Jadelle was first registered in Thailand and Indonesia for up to 3 years' use and was later registered for up to 5 years' use in the USA and in some European countries. It is currently awaiting the outcome of registration applications in a further 30 countries or so.

Implanon is a single-rod system delivering the progestogen etonorgestrel. It is made by the Dutch firm Organon and was first registered in Indonesia in 1998. It has since been registered in over 90 countries.

A third new device is an implant still under development by Population Council researchers that uses a single rod releasing the synthetic progestogen nestorone. This hormone is inactive when ingested orally and is thus particularly suited for use by breastfeeding mothers, whose infants will not be affected by hormone that might be transferred to babies via breast milk.

A fourth device Uniplant (or Surplant) delivers the synthetic progestogen nomegestrol acetate. Because this device offers little or no advantage over other devices, the company holding its patent has shelved plans to market it.

The main difference, of course, between Norplant and the newer implants is the smaller number of rods or capsules in the newer devices, which can therefore be inserted and removed more easily. Largely because of this comparative advantage, the newer implants are expected increasingly to replace Norplant in coming years (Table 6.10).

Under local anesthetic and using a small incision, the implant is inserted under the skin. It is effective within 24 hours of insertion and has a 5-year duration of action with constant release. There are no estrogen-related effects. Removal is possible, following which return to fertility occurs quickly, and the implant is safe, effective, and well-liked.

The woman should, however, be fully counseled. She should be told what side effects to expect and also that she can, and has a right to, have the implant removed at any time, if she is unhappy about the method due to side effects or if she wants the implant removed for other reasons. Side effects are similar to those found with long-acting progestogen-only contraceptives and include irregular bleeding, amenorrhea, and occasional weight change.

Table 6.10 Contraceptive implants, available or being developed

Implant	Distinctive components	Registration	Life span (years)	Percent failure (pregnancy per year)	Chief mechanism of action
Norplant	6 silicone capsules releasing levonorgestrel	In about 60 countries	7[a]	<1	Inhibits ovulation and makes cervical mucus impenetrable by sperm
Jadelle	2 silicone rods releasing levonorgestrel	In some EU countries, USA, Thailand, and Indonesia	5	<1	Inhibits ovulation and makes cervical mucus impenetrable by sperm
Implanon	1 polymer (resin) rod releasing etonogestrel	Over 90 Countries including Australia, Indonesia, USA and many EU countries	3	<1	Suppresses ovulation and endometrial development
Nestorone	1 silicone rod releasing nestorone	In Brazil	2[b]	<1	Suppresses ovulation
	1 silicone capsule releasing nestorone (Elcometrine)		0.5[c]	Not Known	Suppresses ovulation
Uniplant	1 silicone capsule releasing nomegestrol acetate		1	~1	Inhibits ovulation and makes cervical mucus impenetrable by sperm

[a] Approved for 5 years.
[b] Intended life span.
[c] Approved.

The removal procedure takes a little longer than the insertion procedure. Furthermore, the healthcare providers have to be trained properly in both procedures of insertion and removal. The healthcare provider should be trained in counseling and should know that a woman has a right to request removal and that her wishes should be complied with.

Etonogestrel implant (Implanon)

This long-acting reversible hormonal contraceptive implant consists of a single rod containing 68 mg of etonogestrel, releasing a daily amount of around 60–70 µg. It is inserted subdermally in about 1 minute via a specially designed sterile disposable applicator (Figure 6.12).

Implanon acts reliably for a period of 3 years, after which it is recommended that a new implant be inserted provided pregnancy or an alternative method are not desired. Since it is a progesterone-only contraceptive, it has limited side effects and is suitable for use by a wide range of women, including those who cannot use combined hormonal contraceptive methods. Implanon can be used safely and conveniently in women who want to prevent a first pregnancy, as well as those who want some form of 'sterility', albeit easily reversible, until they complete their reproductive years.

The 'patch'

The patch provides daily steroid doses equivalent to the lowest dose oral contraceptives. Its active ingredients are ethinylestradiol and norelgestromin. It has been approved for use by the FDA since 2002, and is gaining popularity due to its relative ease of use and few side effects.

Maximum serum concentrations are lower with the patch than with oral contraceptives because the patch is a sustained-release system. The size of the patch determines daily dose and maximum concentrations.

A new patch should be worn every week for 3 consecutive weeks, followed by a patch-free week. The site where the patch is applied should be changed with each new patch, i.e. every week. Body sites that are recommended for use are the lower abdomen, upper outer arm, buttocks, and upper torso (excluding breasts) (Figure 6.13).

Studies have shown that compliance with the patch is much higher than that with the oral contraceptive pill, probably owing to the fact that changing the patch is a 'once a week' activity, which is much easier than remembering to take a pill every day.

Side effects of the patch are minimal. The only symptom that appears to be more common with its use is breast tenderness. A rare side effect, which is exclusive to the patch, is skin irritation.

Once removed, return to fertility is almost immediate. The overall failure rate is around 1–3%. Similar to the 'missed pill', there are guidelines for the appropriate action to be taken in case of a 'fallen patch', depending on the time since when the patch was dislodged.

Vaginal contraceptive ring

NuvaRing (Organon) is a flexible ethylene vinyl acetate ring that releases etonogestrel and ethinylestradiol in small amounts daily and, once inserted, is left in place for three consecutive weeks followed by a ring-free week where menstruation is expected to occur. It comes in one size which fits all women (Figure 6.15). It is self administered with low side effect and is 99% effectively.

In order to meet the requirements of the UK licensing authorities for registration of the levonorgestrel-releasing

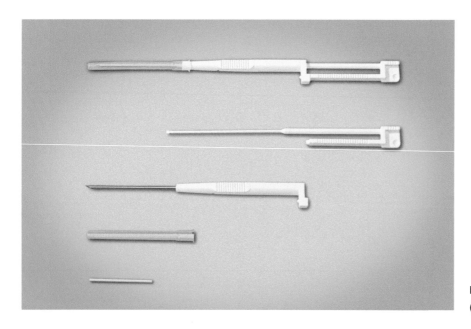

Figure 6.12 Implanon insertion kit. (From reference 22, with permission.)

Wearing the Patch

The contraceptive patch can be worn on four places on your body

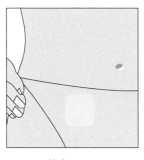
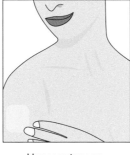
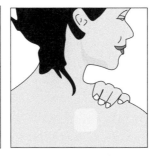
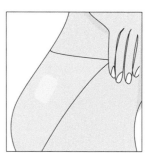

| Abdomen | Upper outer arm | Upper Torso
(front or back, but not your breasts) | Buttocks |

How the patch is used

	Month						
1st patch	1	2	3	4	5	6	7
2nd patch	8	9	10	11	12	13	14
3rd patch	15	16	17	18	19	20	21
No patch	22	23	24	25	26	27	28

Each patch is worn for a 7-day period.
After using three patches in a row,
no patch is worn during the fourth week.

Figure 6.13 The contraceptive patch. (Courtesy of Ortho-McNeil Pharmaceutical, 2001.)

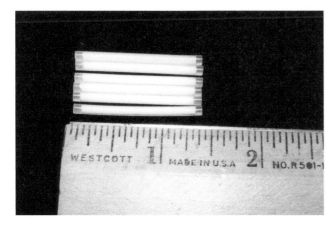

Figure 6.14 An example of a single-use prefilled syringe. It cna be used for long-acting injectable contraceptives (Coutsey of The Program for Applied Technology in Health)

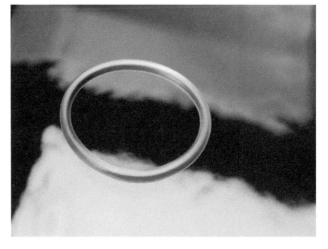

Figure 6.15 The NuvaRing. (From reference 23, with permission.)

vaginal ring developed by HRP, the company licenced to manufacture the rings undertook a phase III clinical trial of machine-manufactured rings in British women. The study confirmed the efficacy of the ring shown in the earlier WHO studies, but also found (in some women) localized lesions of uncertain significance and etiology on the vaginal wall. Since pressure of the ring on the vaginal wall was a possible cause of the lesions, the ring's geometry was modified to increase its flexibility, and research is under way to assess the redesigned ring.

REFERENCES

1. Population Reports, Volume XXVIII, No.1, Spring 2000 Series A, No. 9. Oral Contraceptives.

2. Hatcher RA, Trussel J, Stewart F et al. Contraceptive Technology 17th edn. New York: Ardent Media, 1998: 435.

3. Sharp D. Four up, one back – and no-one off. Lancet 2004; 363: 1252.

4. Wymelenberg S. Science and Babies: Private Decisions, Public Dilemmas. Family Health International. New York: Ballantine Books, 1987.

5. Hankinson SE, Colditz GA, Hunter DJ et al. A quantitative assessment of oral contraceptive use and risk of ovarian cancer. Obstet Gynecol 1992; 80(4): 708–14.

6. Emons G, Fleckenstein G, Hinney B, Huschmand A, Heyl W. Hormonal interactions in endometrial cancer. Endocr Rel Cancer 2000; 7(4): 227–42.

7. Collaborative Group on Hormonal Factors in Breast Cancer. Breast cancer and hormonal contraceptives: collaborative reanalysis of individual data on 53 297 women with breast cancer and 100 239 women without breast cancer from 54 epidemiological studies. Lancet 1996; 347: 1713–27.

8. http://imaginis.com/breasthealth/statistics.asp#1

9. http://www.cancer.gov/cancertopics/factsheet/risk/HPV

10. Franceschi S. The IARC commitment to cancer prevention: The example of papillomavirus and cervical cancer. Recent Results in Cancer Research 2005; 166: 277–97.

11. Smith JS, Green J, Berrington de GA et al. Cervical cancer and use of hormonal contraceptives: a systematic review. Lancet 2003; 361(9364): 1159–67.

12. Moreno V, Bosch FX, Munoz N et al. Effect of oral contraceptives on risk of cervical cancer in women with human papillomavirus infection: the IARC multicentric case-control study. Lancet 2002; 359(9312): 1085–92.

13. Franceschi S. The IARC commitment to cancer prevention: the example of papillomavirus and cervical cancer. Rec Res Cancer Res 2005; 166: 277–97.

14. Yu MC, Yuan JM. Environmental factors and risk for hepatocellular carcinoma. Gastroenterology 2004; 127(5 Suppl 1): S72–8.

15. Expecting a Baby. London: BBC Publications.

16. Himmerick KA. Enhancing contraception: a comprehensive risk. J Am Acad Physician Assist 2005; 18: 26–33.

17. WHO Selected Practice Recommendations Update. Missed pills: new recommendations. Selected Practice Recommendations for Contraceptive Use, 2nd edn. Department of Reproductive Health and Research, Family and Community Health. Geneva: WHO, 2004.

18. Jones RK, Darroch JE, Henshaw SK. Contraceptive use among U.S. women having abortions in 2000–2001. Perspect Sex Reprod Health 2002; 34(6): 294–303.

19. Blumenthal PD, McIntosh N. PocketGuide for Family Planning Service Providers, 2nd edn. Baltimore, Maryland: JHPIE60 Corporation, 1996.

20. Population reports, April 2005, Series M, Number 19, Special Topics.

21. Population Reports, December 2006, Expanding Services for Injectables. How Family Planning Programs and Providers Can Meet Clients' Needs for Injectable Contraceptives, Series K, No. 6. Injectables and Implants.

22. Yong S. A practical approach to contraception and family planning. Implanon Clinician's Manual, Organon. http://www.ncbi.nlm.nih.gov/entrez/query.fcgl?cmd=

23. http://hcp.organon.com

CHAPTER 7

Condoms

Condoms are a commonsense method of contraception with a long history. The 15th century anatomist Gabriel Fallopius, who first described the uterine tubes which still carry his name, described the use of chemically impregnated silk sheaths. His work involved one of the first clinical trials in the history of medicine and, interestingly, he described use of the device after coitus. The word condom is sometimes ascribed to Dr Condom of the Court of Charles II, who was so worried about the number of illegitimate children fathered by the King that he invented the device. This story is probably apocryphal; a more likely derivation of the name is from the Latin 'condus' for 'receptacle'.

Condoms became a widespread family planning method only in the 20th century. Prior to that, they were used principally for the prevention of sexually transmissible infections. An advertisement for condoms in 1796 read:

> To guard yourself from shame or fear,
> Votaries to Venus hasten here,
> None in my ware e'er found a flaw,
> Self-preservation's Nature's law.

Britain appears to have been the first country to commercialize the sale of condoms. Initially, sheaths were made from animal membranes and in the USA 'natural skins' are still sold as luxury items. They are made from the ceca of Australian sheep, removed in the slaughterhouse and cleaned and then shipped to the Caribbean where small elastic rings are sewn into the open ends before they are packaged and sold in the USA.

Rubber condoms became possible after the vulcanization of rubber was first carried out by Hancock and Goodyear in 1844. In the second half of the 19th century hand-dipped devices were made and in the 20th century large-scale mass production (Figure 7.1) and quality control of high-quality rubber condoms (Figure 7.2) were devised. Major manufacturers are in Japan, Taiwan, Western Europe, and the USA.

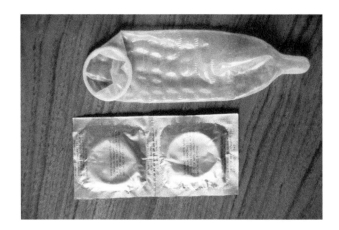

Figure 7.1 An example of a high-quality rubber condom.

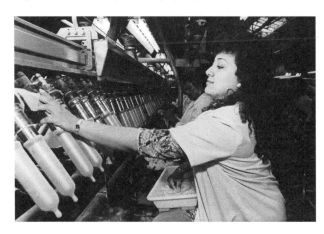

Figure 7.2 Electronic testing of condoms (Durex – London Rubber Company factory).

A relatively small number of manufacturers control production and most of the sales also go through relatively few distributors. Although there are no specific monopolistic practices, new manufacturers find it difficult to break into the market and profit margins are relatively high.

As noted earlier, there are biological reasons why we are all innately shy about human sexual intercourse and therefore

Table 7.1   Use of condoms among married couples of reproductive age in various countries

Region and country	Year	Percent using any method	Percent using condoms
Asia and Pacific			
Bangladesh	2004	58.1	4.2
China	1997	83.8	3.4
Indonesia	2002/03	60.3	0.9
Singapore	1997	62.0	22.0
Thailand	1996/97	72.2	1.8
Latin America and Caribbean			
Brazil	1996	76.7	4.4
Costa Rica	1999	80.0	10.9
El Salvador	2002/03	67.3	2.9
Paraguay	2004	72.8	11.9
Near East and North Africa			
Egypt	2003	60.0	0.9
Iran	1997	72.9	5.4
Turkey	1998	63.9	8.2
Sub-Saharan Africa			
Angola	2001	6.2	0.3
Kenya	2003	39.3	1.2
Nigeria	2003	12.6	1.9
Developed countries			
France	1994	74.6	5.0
Italy	1995/96	60.2	13.7
Japan	2000	55.9	42.1
USA	1995	76.4	13.3

Source: United Nations, Department of Economic and Social Affairs – Population Division: *World Contraceptive Use 2005 – Wall Chart.*

coy about contraception (see Chapter 4). Condoms have long been perceived as a shameful under-the-counter product. One way of defusing embarrassment is through humor; therefore, anthropomorphic penises putting on condoms have become an increasingly widespread educational device, appearing on T-shirts from Sweden to Thailand. Simple illustrations of the correct use of condoms are provided by many organizations around the world. Family Health International owns a 77 000 cubic foot non-lubricated nipple-ended hot-air balloon. For some people it was the ultimate symbol of all that was embarrassing about family planning. It is notable that the *Guinness Book of Records* has never acknowledged an application for its inclusion and North Carolina banned its use. It was accepted in Montreal – providing any written message that it carried was translated into French!

Latex condoms have a limited shelf-life. Contact with oil-based as opposed to aqueous lubricants can greatly weaken a rubber condom within 30 seconds. Even when purchased in bulk, a year's supply of latex condoms is more expensive than oral contraceptives. It is possible to make condoms out of a number of plastics (and they are resistant to oil-based lubricants), but they have not been as aggressively promoted as they might have been.

FAMILY PLANNING

Condoms were the major artificial method of family planning in the UK until the second half of the 20th century and they remain the commonest method in Japan (see Figure 5.5). Table 7.1 shows the use of condoms among couples of reproductive age in a sample of countries. Condoms have no significant side effects. The most common reason for failure is non-use.

Condoms illustrate the difficulty of assessing contraceptive failure rates. The normal measure is the number of pregnancies per 100 woman-years of exposure (e.g. 100 women using the method for 1 year or 20 women for 5 years). There have been relatively few studies of condom use and those that do exist have not been conducted to the exacting standards of modern clinical trials. When couples have used condoms for many years, they often achieve failure rates of well under five pregnancies per 100 woman-years of exposure. However, those who are not familiar with the method make many more mistakes.

When assessing the failure rate of any method of contraception, it is rarely useful to quote an exact number but more informative to give a range of failure rates. It is easy to establish a rank order for effectiveness of methods of contraception

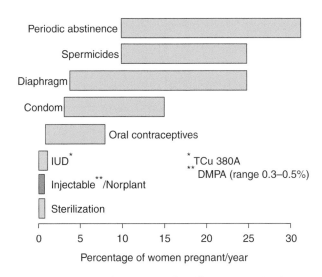

Figure 7.3 Range of failure rates for different methods of contraception. DMPA = depo-medroxyprogesterone acetate.

Table 7.2 The four broad areas in which action needs to be taken to ensure that condoms are used every time they are needed

Promoting condoms to the public
Informing and counseling people so that they may use condoms consistently and correctly
Making condoms universally available at affordable prices
Manufacturing more condoms as demand grows

Table 7.3 Initiatives which should be taken by the policymakers to increase the use of condoms

Eliminate all barriers to import or manufacture, including duties and taxes
Make increasing condom use a top public health priority
Encourage innovative distribution, such as employment-based programs, social marketing programs, community-based distribution, and school-based programs
Eliminate policy and legal barriers to condom promotion

(Figure 7.3), with condoms being more effective than coitus interruptus and oral contraceptives being more effective than condoms. Nevertheless, there will still be people who probably would use the pill less effectively than the condom, and vice versa.

SEXUALLY TRANSMITTED INFECTIONS

For several decades, those working in family planning have tried to separate the use of condoms for contraception from their use for protection against sexually transmitted diseases. With the spread of AIDS, condoms are once again becoming a significant, life saving item. Unfortunately, condom promotion, like many aspects of family planning and AIDS prevention proved easily politicized. Instead of objectively recognizing both the advantages and possible disadvantages of condom use, some politicians and religious leaders have attempted to label condoms as too ineffective to use.

Good-quality latex condoms are impervious to bacteria and viruses, although condoms made from animal membranes are permeable to viruses. Clinical studies show that latex condoms offer substantial protection against herpes simplex, *Chlamydia trachomatis*, cytomegalovirus, *Neisseria gonorrhoeae*, and *Ureaplasma urealyticum*.

Unlike pregnancy, however, sexually transmitted infection can take place at any time in the ovarian cycle and consistent use – as high as 85% of all all sexual acts – is needed to control infections.

It is particularly important when condoms are used to prevent HIV/AIDS to promote a balanced policy of 'ABC': **A**bstinence when possible; **B**e faithful to your partner; and use **C**ondoms when exposed to a risk of infection by HIV or a bacterial infection.

AN OLD DEVICE IN A NEW SETTING

Condoms can prevent unwanted pregnancy and death and morbidity from HIV and other sexually transmitted infections. In developing countries, condom use is constrained more by lack of subsidies to make condoms affordable than by lack of demand. In sub-Saharan Africa the supply of condoms is equivalent to three pieces per adult man per year.

The public health challenge today is therefore to try to ensure that condoms are used each and every time they are needed. This task is not simple, easy, or quick; but it is urgent and important. Action is needed in four broad areas, as indicated in Table 7.2, and in order to increase condom use, policymakers should take the steps illustrated in Table 7.3.

CHAPTER 8

Female barrier contraception and spermicides

BARRIER CONTRACEPTION

In the early 19th century, experiments began with a variety of cervical and vaginal barriers, several of which are in current use. The first-ever written prescription for a contraceptive (barrier method) tampon can be found in the *Ebers Papyrus*, a compendium of medical practices written in 1550 BC. The greatest appeal of barrier methods is also their greatest drawback: they have no apparent effects on the human system and need to be used only at the time of intercourse. However, they are less effective than other methods. They should be used with a spermicide, as this improves effectiveness.

SPERMICIDES

A number of chemicals kill sperm. The most commonly used is nonoxynol-9 (N-9), and most spermicides contain this non-ionic detergent.[1]

Spermicides can be used alone or in combination with a barrier such as a diaphragm (Figure 8.1). Spermicides can be formulated as pessaries, gels, foams from an aerosol can, or in the form of a water-soluble film (Figure 8.2). While spermicides can kill a number of bacterial sexually transmitted diseases, in high doses or in sensitive individuals, spermicides can damage the vaginal epithelium or cause penile irritation, and possibly accelerate the process of transmission of HIV.

Evidence suggests that it is safe for women at low or no risk of HIV to continue to use spermicides containing N-9 for birth control purposes. Women who may be at risk of HIV and who plan to use the product more than once a day should consider switching to another form of birth control.

THE SPONGE

Sponges of various shapes and types have been available for many years. Disposable plastic sponges, such as the Today

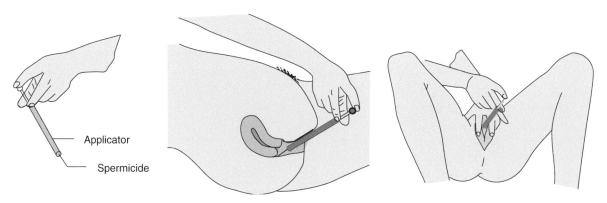

Figure 8.1 Technique of inserting a spermicide.

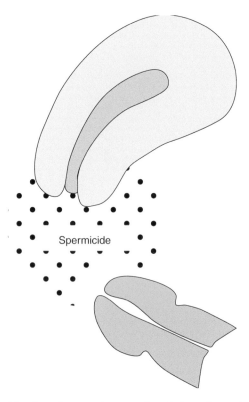

Figure 8.2 Site of action of spermicides which can be used.

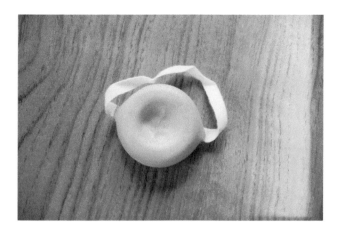

Figure 8.3 Disposable plastic sponge alone or in combination with a barrier.

sponge, impregnated with a spermicide, were first marketed in the 1980s (Figure 8.3).

Today sponge became the largest-selling over-the-counter (OTC) female contraceptive in the United States. It provides women with what they most often look for in a contraceptive: effectiveness, safety, convenience, and sexual spontaneity. Made of a soft, disposable polyurethane foam that feels like natural vaginal tissue, Today sponge contains the widely used spermicide N-9. After it is moistened with water and inserted into the vagina, Today sponge becomes effective immediately and protects against pregnancy for the next 24 hours without the need to add spermicidal cream or jelly – even with repeated acts of intercourse.

The Today sponge was made available in the USA, Canada, and some European countries. In 1984 it was the method of choice for more than 1.2 million women in the USA, about 4% of all US contraceptive users.

The Today sponge was discontinued in 1994, when the producer deemed new US Food and Drug Administration (FDA) manufacturing standards too costly to meet. In 1999, the Allendale Pharmaceutical Company purchased the rights to manufacture the Today sponge and in April 2005 received US FDA approval to market it in the USA. The Today sponge also has been re-released in Canada and is expected to become available elsewhere within several years.

The sponge is less effective than most other methods as commonly used. Among typical users 13–16 women per 100 become pregnant in the first year of use.

Protectaid is a new polyurethane foam sponge that is premoistened and packed with a gel called F-5. The gel contains low concentrations of N-9, sodium cholate, and benzalkonium chloride, along with a dispersal agent that encourages the diffusion of the gel to form a protective coating on the surface of the vagina. The F-5 gel has spermicidal and microbicidal properties. The manufacturer contends that the combination of three spermicides allows use of smaller amounts of each, and this minimizes the risk of irritation of vaginal and cervical tissue.

The Protectaid sponge is available in Canada, China, Egypt, Hong Kong, Israel, Spain, the Ukraine, and the UK. The manufacturer is applying for regulatory approval in other countries and may also apply for US FDA approval.[2]

CERVICAL CAP

The cervical cap was invented in the early 19th century and caps were on sale in New York in the 1860s, but they were not approved by the FDA until the 1980s. The cervical cap is a small thimble-shaped device of rubber or metal that fits directly around the cervix (Figure 8.4). It should form an airtight seal and is held in place by suction. A small quantity of spermicide is applied before insertion, and the cap can be left in position for several days. The cervical cap is held in place by the cervix; thus, sizing the cervix is very critical in fitting a cervical cap. Incorrect sizing of the cervix can lead to dislodgment of the cap during intercourse.

Two new contraceptive cervical caps, FemCap and Oves, are on the market in several countries. Worldwide, few women use cervical caps, in part because they usually require fitting by a provider, and few providers are trained

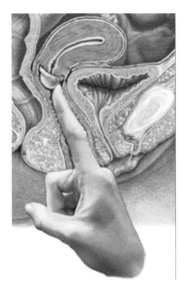

Barrier method: the cervical cap fits snugly over the cervix, preventing sperm from entering the uterus

Figure 8.4 The cervical cap.

in fitting. New cervical caps are designed to reduce fitting time.

Femcap, manufactured by FemCap, Inc., is a silicone rubber device with a dome that fits snugly over the cervix and blocks the passage of sperm. It has been available for several years in Austria, Finland, Germany, Italy, and Switzerland. In 2003 the FDA approved it for use with spermicide. FemCap comes in three sizes: women who have never been pregnant use the smallest size, women who have miscarried, had a termination of pregnancy, or delivered by cesarian section use the medium size; and women who have delivered a full-term baby vaginally use the largest size. Obstetric history predicts the right size about 85% of the time. A provider must still check the fit of the device. In a comparative trial, pregnancy rates among users of the FemCap were significantly higher than those among diaphragm users, but within the range expected for cervical barriers. Pregnancy rates for the FemCap estimated based on this 6-month study are 18 per 100 women per year of use.

FemCap contains a groove on the outside so that users can apply a spermicide, or microbicide once available, to the outside as well as the inside surface of the groove. It also features a brim that forms a seal against the vaginal walls for further protection. FemCap was designed to dislodge less often than other cervical caps and to put less pressure on the urethra than the diaphragm, although there is insufficient research to determine whether FemCap achieves these objectives.

Oves is a disposable cervical cap manufactured by Veos, Ltd., a French company, and first introduced in France in 1997. It is also available in several other European countries and Canada. Oves is made of thin silicone instead of latex, as most diaphragms are. Like FemCap, it comes in three

sizes and must be fitted by a provider. Its effectiveness has not yet been established.

Unlike other caps, Oves does not rely on suction of the cap rim against the cervix. The thin dome of the cap resembles a membrane and adheres to the cervix like a film – a feature intended to make it comfortable and undetectable in use. In acceptability studies women report some difficulty in placing Oves over the cervix and in removing it. Ease of insertion and removal increases with experience, but some women continue to have difficulty removing the cap.[2]

DIAPHRAGMS

The diaphragm is a cervical barrier type of birth control (Figure 8.5). It is a soft latex or silicone dome with a spring molded into the rim. The spring creates a seal against the walls of the vagina. Diaphragms come in different sizes. A fitting appointment with a healthcare professional is necessary to determine which size a woman should wear.

A correctly fitting diaphragm will cover the cervix and rest snugly against the pubic bone. A diaphragm that is too small might fit inside the vagina without covering the cervix, or might become dislodged from the cervix during intercourse or bowel movements. It is also more likely, during intercourse, that a woman's partner will feel the anterior rim of a too-small diaphragm. A diaphragm that is too large will place pressure on the urethra, preventing the bladder from emptying completely and increasing the risk of urinary tract infection.

Diaphragms should be refitted after a weight change of 4.5 kg (10 lb) or more. An increase in weight may cause a

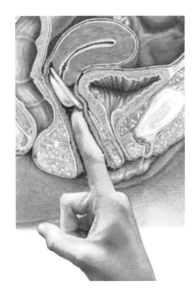

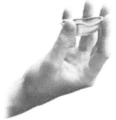

Barrier method: the diaphragm fits over the cervical opening, preventing sperm from entering the uterus

Figure 8.5 Cross-sectional view of the correct positioning of the diaphragm.

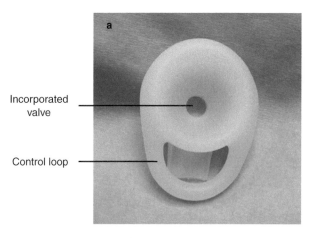
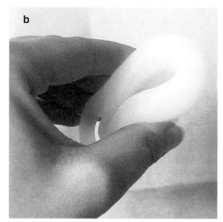

Incorporated valve

Control loop

Figure 8.6   (a) Lea's shield; (b) squeezed.[3] (with kind permission from Yana, Inc., Union, NJ.)

woman to need a smaller diaphragm; a decrease in weight may cause her to need a larger one.

Diaphragms should also be refitted after any pregnancy of 14 weeks or longer. Full-term vaginal delivery especially will tend to increase the size diaphragm a woman needs, although the changes to the pelvic floor during pregnancy mean even women who experience second-trimester miscarriage, or deliver by cesarean section, should be refitted.

Vaginal tenting, an increase in the length of the vagina occurs during arousal. This means that during intercourse, the diaphragm will not fit snugly against the pubic bone – it is carried higher up the vaginal canal by the movement of the cervix. If the diaphragm is inserted after arousal has begun, extra care must be taken to ensure the device is covering the cervix.

A woman might be fitted with a different size diaphragm depending on where she is in her menstrual cycle. It is common for a woman to wear a larger diaphragm during menstruation. It has been speculated that a woman may be fitted with a larger-size diaphragm when she is near ovulation. The correct size for a woman is the largest size that she can wear comfortably throughout her cycle.

Failure rates can be as low as 6% when used with spermicide and under-perfect use. On the other hand failure rates can vary from 10–39% under typical use.

LEA'S SHIELD

Lea's shield is a cup-shaped device made of soft silicone rubber (Figure 8.6). It comes in one size designed to fit most women. The shield is placed over the cervix and features a one-way valve designed to allow air and cervical secretions to pass out, while maintaining a tight fit. The Lea's shield is not held in place by the cervix, but rather by the vagina's wall; therefore, cervix size does not play a role. It also contains a loop at the front end to facilitate removal. It covers the cervix, blocking sperm from reaching the

cervical canal, and has been designed to hold a spermicide or microbicide. It can be reused after washing with soap and water.

The FDA approved Lea's shield for use with a spermicide in 2002. It has been approved in several other countries, including Austria, Canada, Germany, and Switzerland. In the USA, Lea's shield is available by prescription only and costs US$65. The device does not require fitting by a doctor and therefore, in principle, could be made available OTC instead of by prescription.

Data on effectiveness are limited. In a clinical trial among 146 women studied for 6 months, about 9 women per 100 who used Lea's shield with spermicide, and 13 women per 100 who used it without spermicide, became pregnant.

The SILCS intravaginal contraceptive device is a silicone device placed in the vagina to cover the cervix.[2] It has 'grip dimples' on the sides of the rim, and its shape makes insertion and removal easy. The device was developed by PATH and SILCS, Inc., and CONRAD supported product development and clinical trials.

The designers of the device relied heavily on results from studies of current and former diaphragm users and clinicians to improve acceptability and satisfaction. Women are evaluating the new device for comfort and ease of use in studies underway in the Dominican Republic, South Africa, Thailand, and the USA.

FEMALE CONDOMS

The female condom (FC) is a prelubricated strong, soft, transparent sheath that is 17 cm long (about 6.5 inches – the same as a male condom), with a flexible ring at each end. Instead of covering the penis like an ordinary condom, it gently lines the vagina. It is inserted in a similar way to a tampon and is held in place at the upper end of the vagina by a small ring inside the sheath. This does not require precise placement over the cervix. A removable ring helps to insert it as well as keeping

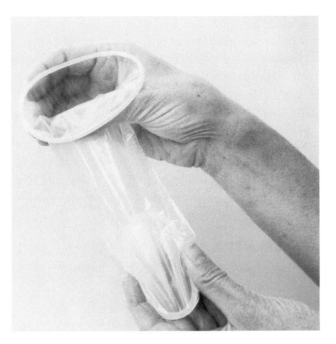

Figure 8.7 The female condom.

the condom in place. A large flexible ring remains on the outside of the vagina, covering the opening of the vagina (vulva) and providing added protection. The first female condom (Figure 8.7) was launched in 1988. A female condom under the trade-name Reality is available in the USA. Like the more traditional male equivalent, the female condom protects against pregnancy and provides a barrier to HIV and other sexually transmissible organisms (Figure 8.8).

This FC was the first widely available condom to be made of polyurethane: a stronger material than latex which, however, is soft and comfortable, allowing a greater degree of sensitivity for many couples. The FC is too costly for many family planning programs or clients. Several newer female condoms – the FC2, the VA feminine condom, and the PATH woman's condom – are made of less costly materials than the FC female condom. They are now in clinical trials.

The FC2 female condom has the same design and instructions for use as the FC female condom. The material has been changed to improve affordability, while maintaining the high quality, reliability, and features of the FC. FC2's

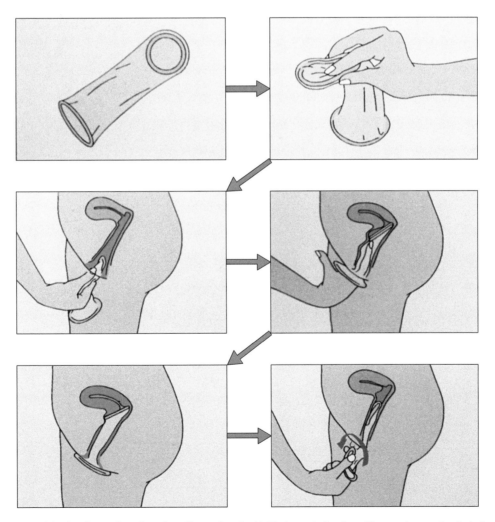

Figure 8.8 Insertion of the female condom, Femidom. (Reproduced with kind permission from Chartex International plc, London, UK.)

sheath, with its outer ring, is made from a synthetic nitrile.The lubricant used is non-spermicidal silicone fluid. Clinical studies have revealed no serious safety issues and there are no reports of allergy to polyurethane or the lubricant. There are no known side effects, unless one is allergic to polyurethane or the lubricant. which is very rare.

Female condoms are very effective when used correctly. This means using a new one every time you have sex. Oil-based lubricant can be used with the female condom. Condoms are for single use only. The female condom *cannot* be used with a male condom because this can cause it to move out of place.[3]

Female condoms are sold for single use, although studies are ongoing of the possible reuse in low-income settings. Studies by the Family Health International and the Reproductive Health Research Unit of the University of Witwatersrand, South Africa, have found that the female condom can be washed up to eight times without compromising the structural integrity.[4,5] WHO recommends use of a new male or female condom for every act of intercourse, where there is a risk of unintended pregnancy and/or STI/HIV infection. Recognizing the urgent need for risk-reduction strategies for women who cannot or do not access new condoms, WHO has developed a protocol for the safe handling and preparation of a used (original) FC female condom that is intended for reuse. WHO does not recommend or promote reuse, but has made available the protocol, together with guidelines on programmatic issues, to program managers who intend to evaluate the feasibility of reuse and application in local settings.

A consensus statement by a WHO expert panel (2002) stated that the female condom could be satisfactorily disinfected, cleaned, and reused up to five times provided that this process was performed according to a specific set of standards, which dictate that the condom should be soaked in 1:20 dilution of sodium hypochlorite (household bleach) for 2–5 minutes prior to washing with soap and water.[5]

REFERENCES

1. Euro. J Contracept Reprod Health Care 2002; 7(3): 173–7.
2. Population Reports' New Contraceptive Choices, Series M, No. 19, April, 2005.
3. Women's Health Information Centre (RWH), The Royal Women's Hospital, Victoria, Australia. FPA Health: http://www.rwh.org.au/womensinfo/factsheets.cfm?doc_id=6126
4. Family Health International. Female condom re-use examined. Health Bull Netw 2000; 20(2).
5. Reuse: Report of a WHO Consultation (January 2002). WHO information update: considerations regarding Reuse of the Female Condom (July 2002). Department of Reproductive Health and Research (RHR), World Health Organization: www.who.int/reproductive-health/rtis/reuse.en.html
6. Supplements to No. 19, April, 2005.

CHAPTER 9

Intrauterine devices

As the need for fertility control grew at the end of the 19th century, important innovations in contraception occurred. The first was the development of the intrauterine device (IUD). IUDs were derived from stem pessaries, which were conceived as devices rather like over-large drawing pins (thumb tacks) designed to prevent the ascent of sperm through the cervix (Figure 9.1). In order to hold them in place, a Y-shaped metal extension was inserted in the uterus. It was observed that, even when the cervical device broke off, the intrauterine metallic portion still exerted a contraceptive effect.

Even to this day there is some dispute over how IUDs work; their effect may be through a number of complementary mechanisms which include changing the uterine environment in order to make implantation of the fertilized egg impossible, as well as reducing the number and motility of sperm reaching the Fallopian tubes and perhaps bringing about changes in tubal physiology; ovum transport and embryo formation may also be affected. The main clinical advantages and disadvantages of IUDs were well understood by the first decade of the 20th century. The devices were widely used by Gräfenberg and others in Europe between the two World Wars. As with many methods of contraception, they can be highly effective (98%) and acceptable, but they also have important limitations and strong contraindications.

An IUD gives long-term, easily reversible, coitally independent contraceptive protection; it does not require continuous motivation for effective use. The plastic IUDs introduced in the 1960s were associated with heavier menstruation and an increased risk of uterine infection in women exposed to sexually transmitted infections. It was observed that the larger the size of the IUD, the lower the failure rate, but the greater the side effects. The addition of

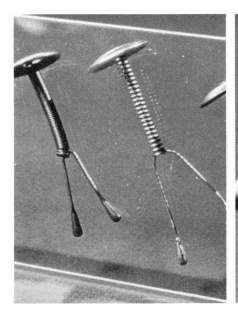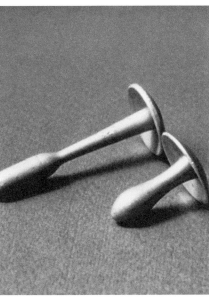

Figure 9.1 Early IUDs. Forerunners of the intrauterine device were the intracervical stems (right) and wishbone intracervical device (left). The stems were sutured to the uterine wall via the small hole in the rim. The wishbone devices were placed in the cervix and the stem protruded into the uterus. (Reproduced with kind permission from Ortho-McNeil Inc., Canada.)

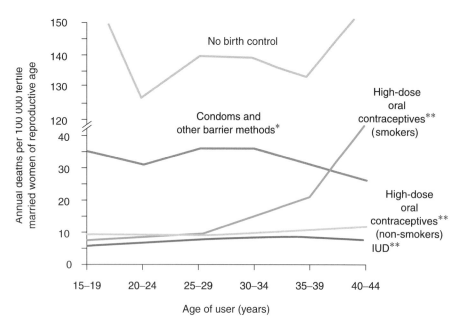

Figure 9.2 Mortality from intrauterine devices compared with other reversible methods and no birth control. Estimated annual deaths resulting from pregnancy, childbirth, contraceptive use, and unintended pregnancy following contraceptive failure, by age of women in low-income developing countries. *, Pregnancy-related deaths; **, method and pregnancy-related deaths. (From reference 1 with permission.)

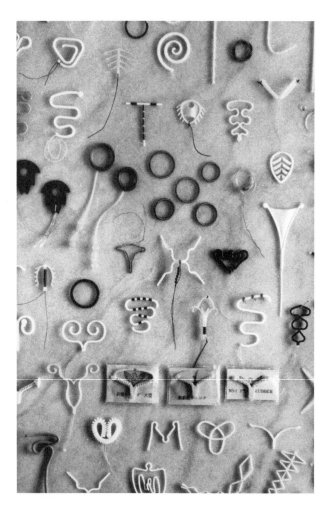

Figure 9.3 An assortment of intrauterine devices.

copper to a device, an invention of Jaime Zipper in Chile, broke this equation and gave a device with fewer side effects and a failure rate of less than two in 100 woman-years of exposure. The third generation of hormone-releasing IUDs both control the bleeding and greatly reduce any increased risk of infection. The idea of drug delivery via IUDs was put forward by Leonard Laufe in North Carolina in 1974, and brought to fruition by Tapani Luukainen of Finland, who developed the levonorgestrol-releasing IUD now sold under the brand name Mirena.

The levonorgestrel-releasing IUD has an even lower failure rate, comparable to that of surgical sterilization. IUDs must be inserted and removed by trained health workers (although not necessarily a physican) under strict aseptic conditions. Women should be counseled about the possibility of pain and discomfort after insertion, changes in menstruation, and to be vigilant about possible infection. IUDs should not be used in women who have multiple sexual partners or whose partners have multiple partners. An alternative method of contraception should be recommended in the presence of acute or chronic pelvic inflammatory disease, known or suspected pregnancy, abnormal uterine bleeding, malignancy of the genital tract, and abnormalities of the uterine cavity. Figure 9.2 shows the mortality from IUDs compared with other reversible methods and no birth control. Uterine perforation is possible and usually takes place during insertion, even though it may not be recognized until later. Perforation is more common postpartum and after second-trimester abortion when the uterus is soft, or during lactation. IUDs can be inserted

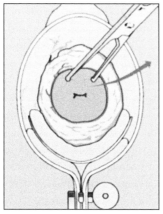

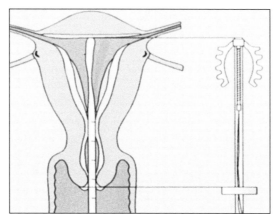

1. Grasp the anterior lip of the cervix with a tenaculum, taking a good bite, and apply steady downward traction, thereby straightening the uterine axis.

2. Straightening of the uterus facilitates sounding and Multiload insertion. Use the sound to measure uterine depth and to confirm the uterine axis, Set the cervical stop of the Multiload at the correct length. This procedure minimizes the risk of perforation and subendometrial insertion.

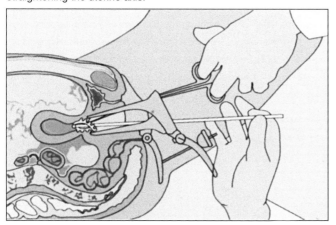

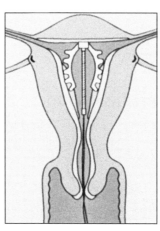

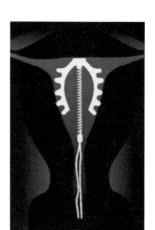

3. No loading procedure is required. During insertion the flexible arms fold back, accommodating to the shape of the cervical canal. Gently push the Multiload into place until it touches the fundus and the cervical stop rests against the external os.
The inserter tube can now be withdrawn. For the actual insertion, only one hand is needed, leaving the other hand free to apply cervical traction during the entire proedure.

4. Trim the threads, leaving 3–4 cm, remove the tenaculum and the speculum. The Multiload now provides reliable, convenient contraception.

Figure 9.4   The insertion of one type of intrauterine device. (Reproduced with kind permission of Organon.)

any time in the menstrual cycle and special techniques are available for immediate (within 30 minutes) insertion after the delivery of the placenta.

Figure 9.3 shows several types of IUD, and Figure 9.4 illustrates the insertion of one such example.

In the early 1970s, by a sad quirk of history, major improvements in IUDs (in particular the addition of copper), together with a good epidemiological understanding of proven side effects, occurred at the very time that the AH Robins Company made major and serious mistakes with the Dalkon Shield. It is characteristic of nearly all methods of contraception that their acceptability and pregnancy rates

are reported to be lowest in carefully supervised clinical trials. In the case of the Dalkon Shield, some of the early users also inserted spermicides around the time of ovulation and the published failure rates were unrealistically low, although this double protection was not explicitly mentioned in relevant publications. Cases of serious pelvic infection occurred (the multifilament thread on the device probably served as wick for bacteria to ascend into the uterine cavity); women who became pregnant with the device in place became seriously ill and some women died as a result of using a Dalkon Shield. AH Robins sought bankruptcy protection and, more importantly, from the point of view of health of women, unreasonable suspicion and pessimism fell on all other IUDs. Even over 30 years later, IUDs remain much less widely used in the USA than their profile as an excellent contraceptive would justify. IUDs remain the most common single method of contraception in the People's Republic of China. Globally, 60 million women use them; of these, only 1.4 million are used by US women and 600 000 by UK women.

EMERGENCY CONTRACEPTION AND IUDs

Effective postcoital contraception can be achieved by the insertion of a copper-containing IUD (see Figure 9.4) within 5 days of unprotected sexual intercourse, and there is some evidence that IUDs are effective when inserted even later. This method may be used when there is a need for continuing contraception and/or where there is a contra-indication for use of the pill postcoitally. Special care should be taken when providing IUDs postcoitally, especially if the client is at risk of pelvic inflammatory disease.

LEVONORGESTREL-RELEASING IUDs

As noted, the levonorgestrel-releasing IUD combine several of the positive characteristics of oral contraceptives, IUDs, and steroid-releasing implants. They largely overcome the drawback of increased menstrual loss associated with inert and even copper IUDs, and the prostestin released by the IUD makes the cervical mucus not only hostile to sperm but also resistant to ascending infections. Levonorgestrel-releasing IUDs also offer an alternative to hysterectomy for some women with menorrhagia at the menopause, and they have been used with hormone replacement therapy (HRT) to overcome the need to use a systemic progestin as well as an estrogen in HRT. Levo-Nova (registered in Finland) and Mirena (registered in the UK and North America) have a daily release of 20 μg levonorgestrel and an estimated effective life of up to 7 years. The main drawback of the levonorgestrel-releasing IUDs is their cost. Unlike oral contraceptives, which depend on the skill and investment of commercial pharmaceutical companies for their continued development, nearly all the development work with levonorgestrel-releasing IUDs was conducted in the not-for-profit sector. However, the cost to the consumer is approximately 100 times their estimated cost of manufacture. High cost prevents these potentially lifesaving devices from being used in low-income settings. Now that the primary patent has expired, it is to be hoped that generic devices will be developed and sold.

REFERENCE

1. Sciarri JJ, Zatuchni J, Speidel. Risks, Benefits and Controversies in Fertility Control. Hagerstown, Maryland: Harper & Row, 1977.

CHAPTER 10

Periodic abstinence and coitus interruptus

Until the early 20th century it was believed that women were maximally fertile at the time of menstruation. In the 1930s Ogino and Knaus demonstrated that ovulation occurs 14 days before the next menstrual period, and soon efforts were made to develop a method of family planning using this information. The rhythm or calendar method is based on predicting the time of ovulation solely on the basis of the length of previous cycles.[1]

One of the effects of estrogen is alteration of the cervical mucus from a thick, opaque sticky consistency to a thin, clear lubricant substance close to the time of ovulation. Progesterone produces a rise in basal body temperature after ovulation. In the basal body temperature method, the woman records her temperature on waking each morning to establish the basal reading; a rise of 0.2–0.4°C occurs at ovulation and the higher reading persists until the onset of menstruation (Figure 10.1). Because of the limited life of the ovum (it can be fertilized for only about 12 hours after release), the woman waits until 3 consecutive days of recording at the higher temperature and can then start intercourse with little risk of conception. Because sperm can survive for up to 3 days, intercourse must be avoided in the

first part of the cycle between menstruation and ovulation (the basal body temperature method cannot predict ovulation), although for part of that time the woman will be infertile. This method requires a long time of abstinence in each cycle but has a high degree of reliability, the rate of unexpected pregnancies varying from less than one to about 6/100 woman-years of use. It is not, however, a practical method for women with very irregular cycles (Table 10.1 and Figures 10.2 and 10.3)

CERVICAL MUCUS

The cervical mucus method involves observation, both by sensation and visual inspection, of the texture of mucus which appears at the vulva. There may be a number of 'dry days' following menstruation (G mucus); thereafter, with rising estrogen levels, the mucus becomes thick and sticky (L-mucus) and then progressively thin, clear, and slippery until the 'peak' day, after which it again changes (S mucus) (Figure 10.4). Abstinence is necessary from the time the mucus appears until the 4th day after peak, when intercourse can be resumed and continued as often as desired until the

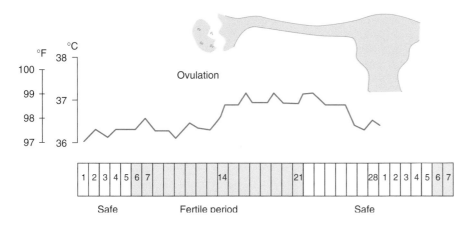

Figure 10.1 The basal body temperature method of periodic abstinence uses temperature recordings throughout the menstrual cycle; a rise of 0.2–0.4°C occurs at ovulation and persists until the onset of menstruation.

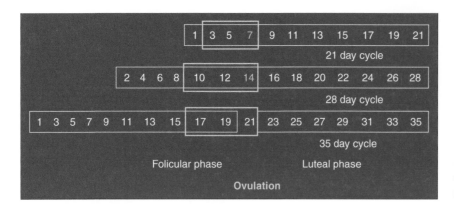

Figure 10.2 Illustration of safe period in women with menstrual cycles of varying lengths. (From reference 2, with permission.)

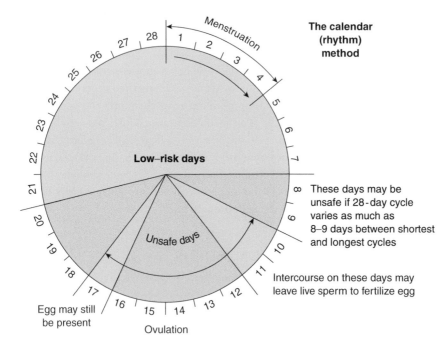

Figure 10.3 Calendar (rhythm) method.[3] (From reference 2, with permission.)

Table 10.1 Calculating the safe period in women with menstrual cycles of varying lengths

Shortest cycle (days)	First unsafe day (−18) after beginning of cycle	Longest cycle (days)	Last unsafe day (−11) after beginning of cycle
21	3rd	21	10th
22	4th	22	11th
23	5th	23	12th
24	6th	24	13th
25	7th	25	14th
26	8th	26	15th
27	9th	27	16th
28	10th	28	17th
29	11th	29	18th
30	12th	30	19th
31	13th	31	20th
32	14th	32	21st
33	15th	33	22nd
34	16th	34	23rd
35	17th	35	24th
36	18th	36	25th

Reproduced from reference 2 with permission.
See also Figure 10.2.

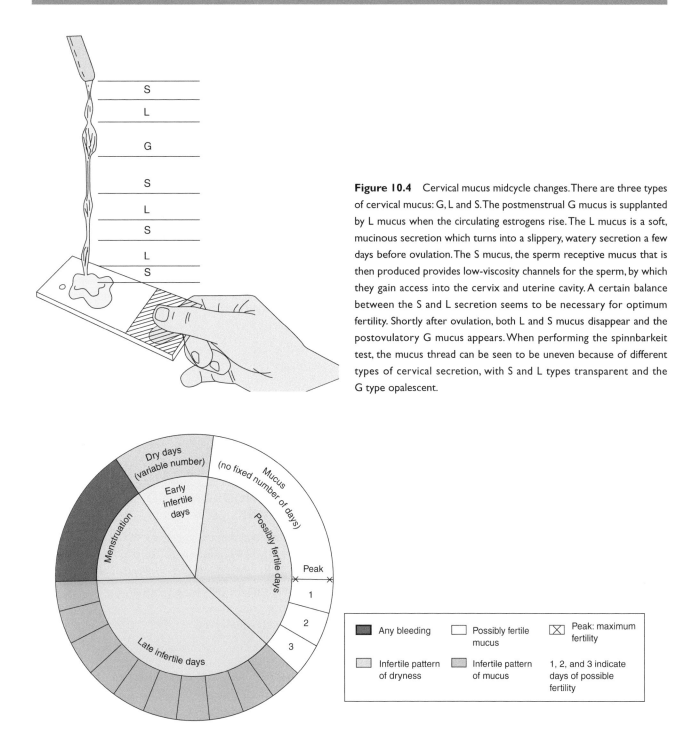

Figure 10.4 Cervical mucus midcycle changes. There are three types of cervical mucus: G, L and S. The postmenstrual G mucus is supplanted by L mucus when the circulating estrogens rise. The L mucus is a soft, mucinous secretion which turns into a slippery, watery secretion a few days before ovulation. The S mucus, the sperm receptive mucus that is then produced provides low-viscosity channels for the sperm, by which they gain access into the cervix and uterine cavity. A certain balance between the S and L secretion seems to be necessary for optimum fertility. Shortly after ovulation, both L and S mucus disappear and the postovulatory G mucus appears. When performing the spinnbarkeit test, the mucus thread can be seen to be uneven because of different types of cervical secretion, with S and L types transparent and the G type opalescent.

Figure 10.5 The mucus pattern of fertility and infertility during the menstrual cycle (peak indicates maximum fertility).

next menstrual period. The duration of abstinence is shorter by this method than by the basal body temperature technique; however, the frequency of unexpected pregnancies is higher, from five to 35/100 woman-years. A 'symptothermal' method combines these two methods of periodic abstinence, and wide variations in the pregnancy rate have been reported – from four to 26 per 100 woman-years. Ovulation methods

need to be carefully tested, but once a couple have learnt the techniques of ovulation prediction, and have the motivation and discipline to practice abstinence when required, no further inputs are needed. Unintended pregnancies, however, sometimes occur during the learning phase.

The identification of the fertile phase can be combined with the use of a barrier method only during those days

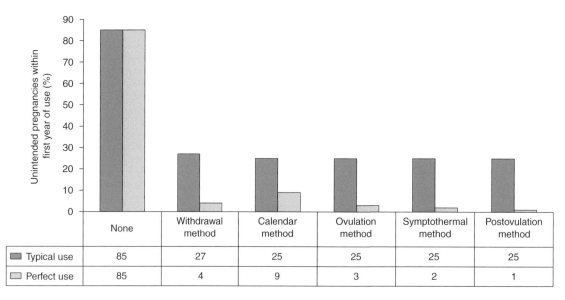

	None	Withdrawal method	Calendar method	Ovulation method	Symptothermal method	Postovulation method
■ Typical use	85	27	25	25	25	25
□ Perfect use	85	4	9	3	2	1

Figure 10.6 A comparison of pregnancy rates using different types of natural methods of contraception. (From reference 4, with permission.)

estimated to be the fertile phase of the woman's cycle (Figure 10.5). Recognition of the time of ovulation is also useful for women seeking to become pregnant, especially if some degree of infertility exists. Self-palpation of the cervix, which softens as ovulation approaches, is another method of timing of periodic abstinence; however, its efficacy has not yet been determined.

Many family planning clients find periodic abstinence more difficult to use than many other methods. Nevertheless, it is better than no method at all (Figure 10.6) and may be the only choice for some individuals and couples. The chart (Figure 10.6) illustrates the risk levels of the specified natural family planning methods for both correct and typical use during the first year, for which data are available.

As is evident from Figure 10.6, both coitus interruptus and periodic abstinence are ineffective by modern standards. Both are superior to the risk of pregnancy (85%) in the first year when no method of contraception is used. Unintended pregnancies among women practicing natural family planning methods are primarily related to user error. Couples who do not use their method correctly – i.e., they have intercourse on days when the method's guidelines tell them that the woman is fertile – have a much greater chance of unintended pregnancy.

No contraception method is both 100% effective and totally free of side effects. The choice of family planning method requires a trade-off between the desired level of protection against pregnancy and the client's willingness to tolerate the risks and disadvantages associated with a particular method. The level of protection from conception is a function of the method itself and how consistently and correctly it is used. The perceived disadvantages of certain methods can often be overcome or alleviated with

appropriate counseling. Interestingly, Saint Augustine condemned the use of what today we would call the rhythm or periodic abstinence method of family planning; despite the early condemnation by theologians, the method has become the only one formally approved in recent Papal encyclicals.

NEW METHODS BASED ON FERTILITY AWARENESS

Two new methods have been developed to help women track their fertile periods. Both methods have been developed by the Institute for Reproductive Health at Georgetown University, with support from USAID:[5]

- Standard Days Method[6]
- Cycle Beads.

CycleBeads and Standard Days are trademarks of Georgetown University. CycleBeads (Figure 10.7) are a patented product and are used by Cycle Technologies under license. Website located at www.cyclebeads.com.

CycleBeads are an easy way to use a natural family planning method. They make it simple for a woman to track her cycle and clearly identify the days she could become pregnant and the days when pregnancy is most unlikely. CycleBeads are based on a natural family planning method that is more than 95% effective when used correctly. They are easy to use, highly effective, and inexpensive, cause no side effects, and can be used to either plan or prevent pregnancy.

CycleBeads make natural family planning easy. To use CycleBeads a woman simply moves a ring over a series of color-coded beads that represent her fertile and low-fertility

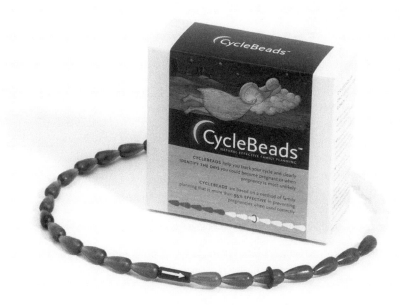

Figure 10.7 CycleBeads.

days. The color of the beads lets her know whether she is on a day when she is likely to be fertile or not.

Use CycleBeads to plan or prevent pregnancy. CycleBeads can be used to achieve pregnancy or avoid pregnancy, depending on the needs of the woman using them. To achieve pregnancy, a woman and her partner can easily determine which days she is most likely to become pregnant. To avoid pregnancy, a woman and her partner can choose to either use another method or not have intercourse on fertile days.

COITUS INTERRUPTUS

The practice of contraception is one of the factors that distinguishes us from other animals: chimpanzees use tools, albeit simple ones, and can be taught a sign language, but, as a theologian observed long ago, we are the only animal that consciously controls our fertility. Perhaps, instead of calling ourselves *Homo sapiens* (the 'wise' man), we should call ourselves *Homo contraceptus*. As noted, coitus interruptus not only has an ancient lineage but also its simplicity and anonymity made it the commonest method of family planning throughout much of Western Europe and the rest of the world. Advantages include the fact that this method is always available, at no cost; however, the failure rate is high, and withdrawal may not always be in time! It is also recommended that the penis is wiped clear of preejaculatory fluid prior to penetration, and this factor may be forgotten by many (Figure 10.8). The data that are available on failure rates suggest they overlap with those of

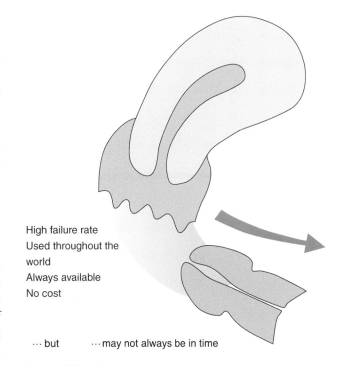

High failure rate
Used throughout the world
Always available
No cost

··· but ···may not always be in time

Figure 10.8 Coitus interruptus.

condoms and mechanical methods. As long ago as the 16th century, Saint Bernadine of Sienna wrote, 'Of one thousand marriages I believe 990 are the devil's', that is, were using coitus interruptus.

As part of the medicalization of fertility regulation, coitus interruptus has come in for some fanciful criticisms, including the possibility of physical and psychological damage. The reality is that human sexual behavior is highly malleable and if a couple love one another they can express that love through coitus interruptus. Coitus interruptus may have become widespread in the West as a result of the criticism of the Church and explicit questions which have been asked for hundreds of years in the confessional. To the ancient Jews and early Christians, semen was a perfect whole and the male was thought to plant his 'seed' in the female, who was not understood to make any contribution to the next generation. By the time of the Prophet Mohammed, the anatomy and physiology of the ovaries were beginning to be understood and it was appreciated that women made a contribution to procreation; and therefore, semen became incomplete. Masturbation and coitus interruptus became less reprehensible. In some contemporary countries, such as Turkey, coitus interruptus remains the major method of contraception and is becoming increasingly common as fertility declines.

REFERENCES

1. Hume K. Fertility awareness in the 1990s – the Billings Ovulation Method of natural family planning, its scientific basis, practical application and effectiveness. Adv Contracept (1991); 7: 301–11.

2. Byer CO, Shainberg LW, Galliano CO. Magnus Hirschfeld Archive for Sexology – methods of contraception. In: Dimensions of Human Sexuality, 5th edn. New York: McGraw-Hill, 1999.

3. Billings JJ, Byer CO, Shainberg LW, Galliano G. In: Archive for sexology Magnus Hirschfeld – Methods of Contraception. In: Dimensions of Human Sexuality, 5th edn. New York: McGraw-Hill, 1999. Med J Aust 1978; 2: 436.

4. Hatcher RA, Trussell JA, Stewart F et al. eds. Contraceptive Technology, 18th edn. New York: Bridging the Gap Communications, 2004.

5. Population Reports, New Contraceptive Choices Series M, No. 19, Special Topics, April 2005. Baltimore, Maryland: INFO Project, Center for Communication Programs, the Johns Hopkins Bloomberg School of Public Health.

6. Arevalo M. Jennings V, Sinai I. Efficacy of a new method of family planning: the Standard Days Method. Contraception 2002; 65: 333–8.

CHAPTER 11

Voluntary surgical contraception

In the USA, voluntary surgical contraception is the single most common modality of family planning. The reality is that even though there is now a wide choice of satisfactory modern methods of contraception, failure of the methods and, more importantly, human errors in use, are sufficiently common that over a fertile lifetime a significant number of couples will have one or more unwanted pregnancies. Any community which is striving to have a small family size must either accept the limitations of reversible methods and be prepared to back them up with safe abortion, or offer a choice of voluntary surgical contraception. Wherever this choice has been made available, it has become an increasingly important part of the family planning choices. As noted in Chapter 9, the failure rate of levonorgestrel-releasing intrauterine devices (IUDs) overlaps with that of surgical sterilization, but underutilization of IUDs in the USA and the high cost of these devices in developing countries prevent the large-scale use of this alternative to surgery.

Voluntary surgical contraception is common in a number of developing countries where fertility has declined rapidly, such as Thailand and Colombia. Where it has been available for several decades, as in the USA, Korea, or the UK, both male and female operations are performed in large numbers. It is common, however, for female sterilization to be offered before male, often beginning with women who have genuine medical contraindications to additional pregnancies, such as diabetes. Female sterilization also makes particular sense to women who have so much more to invest in pregnancy and bringing up children than men, as well as the fact that sterilization in some ways merely represents bringing the infertility aspect of the menopause forward by some years.

Voluntary surgical contraception appears to be attractive to many people in a variety of cultures. Where it is poorly used it is not stopped so much by lack of need, as by a lack of a medical tradition to make the operation available.

Voluntary surgical contraception needs to be made available to all who are definite that they want no more children and who understand the nature of the operation. The operation also needs to be a choice for men and women who have genetic reasons to avoid having children and to women who suffer from serious diseases, such as untreated mitral stenosis. Sterilization, male or female, is usually the most effective method of contraception. Both male and female surgical sterilization have a failure rate, but it is lower than reversible methods of contraception, with the possible exception of hormone-releasing IUDs. Voluntary sterilization is a one-time procedure which is relatively simple in either sex. It does not require constant use of a method or a check-up at regular intervals or the cost of contraceptive supplies. Vasectomy is even simpler than female sterilization. The risk of complications associated with sterilization is minimal if the procedure is performed to strict medical standards. Sterilization operations usually demand a greater degree of skill, training, and equipment than temporary methods of contraception, but they have been safely and responsibly performed by non-physicians in Thailand and elsewhere. Sterilization often gives many years of protection against pregnancy and therefore is amongst the most cost-effective methods of family planning. Table 11.1 outlines the advantages and disadvantages of surgical sterilization.

ETHICAL AND LEGAL ISSUES

Sterilization should always be a voluntary informed choice. A couple should know that all surgery carries with it an irreducible minimum of complications and that the reversal of both male and female sterilization, while it can be attempted sometimes, is always difficult and commonly disappointing in its outcome.

In a few cases – fortunately more talked about than implemented – the state has tried to make sterilization

Table 11.1 Advantages and disadvantages of voluntary surgical contraception

Female sterilization

- The effect is immediate, but there is no way of judging the effectiveness of the procedure
- Postoperative recovery is rapid (ambulatory after a few to 48 hours) and a hospital stay of only 12–48 hours as necessary
- The operation can be classified as an outpatient procedure
- The procedure can be performed under local anesthesia (minimal risk); if general anesthesia is necessary then the risks associated with this apply
- Reversal of the procedure is successful in up to 75% of cases, depending on the particular method of sterilization. However, there is a risk of ectopic pregnancy following reversal
- The operation provides an opportunity to explore the pelvic cavity for gynecological problems. However, there may be operative risk to other organs
- The risk of ovarian cancer is reduced

Vasectomy

- The operation is quick, easy, and safe
- Two negative sperm counts assume sterility, but repeat visits for sperm counts are necessary, 15–30 postoperative ejaculations being needed before sterility occurs
- The operation can be classified as an outpatient procedure
- The procedure can be performed under local anesthesia, which is associated with minimal risk
- Reversal of the procedure is easier as compared with that of female sterilization, provided that the reversal is carried out fairly soon after vasectomy

compulsory under certain circumstances. In the USA, some states passed coercive sterilization laws in the first half of the 20th century, although they have now all been repealed. In 1976, the Maharashtra State in India passed a law imposing fines and imprisonment on anyone with three or more children who refused to be sterilized. The law, however, was never ratified or implemented. There have been reports of coercive sterilization in China, although this was never part of the government one-child policy. Incidentally, no one in India has ever received a transistor radio for a vasectomy – it was suggested by an enthusiastic administrator but was never put into practice. Some countries, such as Bangladesh and Sri Lanka, have given a small monetary compensation or gift such as a sari to those coming for sterilization. Some people have interpreted this as an 'incentive,' while others have claimed it to be a compensation for time lost when very poor people go for surgery.

Anything which changes sterilization from an informed voluntary choice is, and must continue to be, condemned. But it is also important to recognize that non-evidence-based restrictions on access to contraception and voluntary sterilization can lead to what can only be called 'coercive pregnancy.' In many countries, sterilization has been or

remains illegal. Sterilization was never against the law in Britain, although vasectomy did not become part of comprehensive services until 1979. In the middle of the 20th century in the USA, physicians often imposed a '120 rule': i.e the woman's age multiplied by the number of her children had to equal 120 before she was permitted to have a sterilization. Indonesian physicians reinvented this rule in the 1970s. In Brazil, sterilization became routine after three cesarean operations, so that today the majority of all deliveries among rich women are by cesarean section. Human reproduction is too important and too complicated to submit to simple 120 rules and women should not be subjected to unnecessary cesarean operations as a backdoor way of making decisions about family size.

VASECTOMY

Vasectomy (male sterilization) has had a chequered history, beginning in the late 19th century with charlatans who claimed that vasectomy led to male rejuvenation. The operation that is usually practiced today was perfected in India in the 1950s. It is a simple 5-minute procedure performed under a local anesthetic during which the vas deferens is isolated, ligated, and the two ends tied or the lumen cauterized (Figures 11.1–11.4). The key to success is for the surgeon to identify and fix the vas with his fingers prior to surgery. The operation can even be performed through a single, tiny incision using a sharp forceps – the 'no-scalpel' vasectomy, developed by Dr Li Shungiang in China, which has now entered widespread use. As in routine vasectomy, the vas is palpated below the skin of the scrotum. The skin is then perforated with a special pair of forceps. The vas is extracted and occluded. The method is slightly more difficult to learn but is associated with less bleeding and the puncture wound in the skin is so slight that no suture is needed.

Possible complications of vasectomy include the rare possibility of a vasovagal attack, pain, bleeding with hematoma, infection, sinus formation, sperm granuloma, and failure. Vasectomy is not immediately effective. The client has to use condoms or his partner another temporary method until he has had 15–30 ejaculations after vasectomy or until sperm-free semen is demonstrated using semen analysis.

Vasectomy is not recommended as the best method of contraception if the man has a history of impotence or if he has a psychological fear of the procedure or its consequences; or if the wife requires hysterectomy for any reason; or if the marriage faces problems.

FEMALE STERILIZATION

Female sterilization, which requires tubal occlusion using one of a variety of techniques, including surgery, electrocautery,

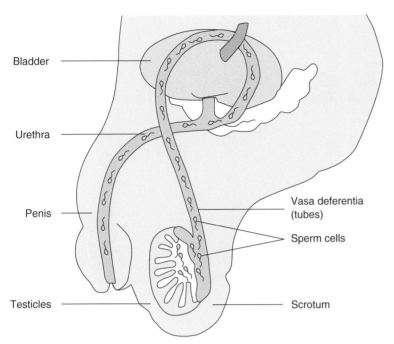

Bladder

Urethra

Penis

Vasa deferentia
(tubes)

Sperm cells

Testicles

Scrotum

Figure 11.1 Lateral view of the male reproductive organs illustrating how the sperm pass freely through the male reproductive tract.

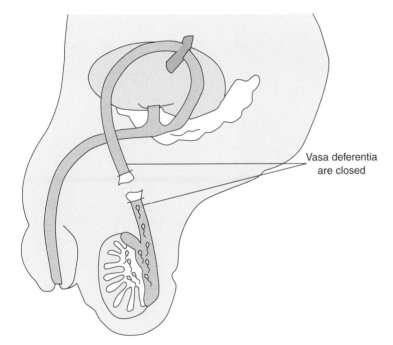

Vasa deferentia
are closed

Figure 11.2 Lateral view of the male reproductive organs illustrating how, after vasectomy, the vasa deferentia are blocked, and sperm cells are prevented from reaching and joining female egg cells.

and the application of clips and rings, necessitates opening the abdominal cavity (Figure 11.5). It is always going to be a more complicated procedure than the male operation. Nevertheless, there have been some remarkable simplifications of technology in the past 30 years, particularly the use of the so-called minilaparotomy where the Fallopian tubes are occluded through an abdominal incision measuring 2–5 cm, and which is usually carried out using a local anesthetic and light sedation. Sterilization can also be performed under local anesthesia

using a laparoscope to locate and occlude the tubes. It has been dubbed the 'band-aid' operation, and can be done on a day-care basis. A variety of mechanical clips, including the Filshie Clip (Figure 11.6) and rings, have been devised; they can be placed with a laparoscope. Clips do minimal damage to the Fallopian tube, making the possibility of repair more likely should the need arise. Electrocautery can also be used but destroys much more of the Fallopian tube. Cautery has an even lower failure rate than clips or rings. Complications of

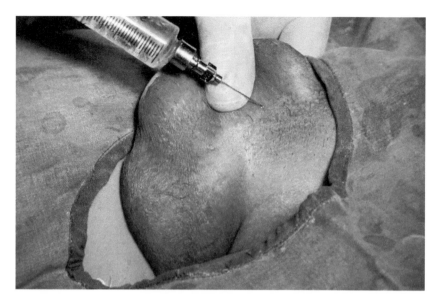

Figure 11.3 Modern vasectomy is a simple procedure which can be done under local anesthesia.

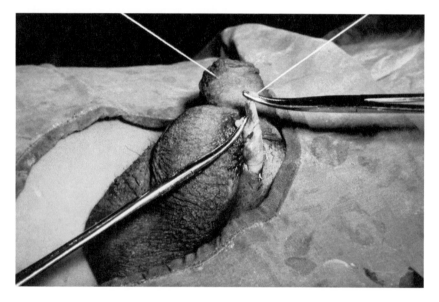

Figure 11.4 Vasectomy: the vas deferens is isolated and ligated.

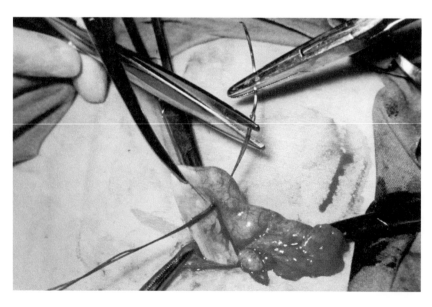

Figure 11.5 Female sterilization: the abdomen is opened through small incisions and the Fallopian tubes are isolated and occluded.

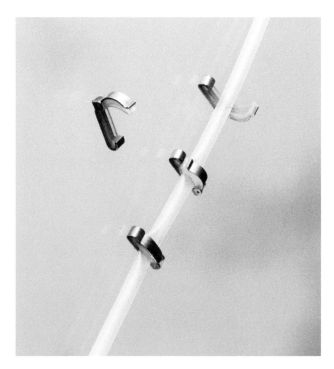

Figure 11.6 Filshie Clip. (Reproduced with kind permission from Femcare Ltd, Nottingham, England.)

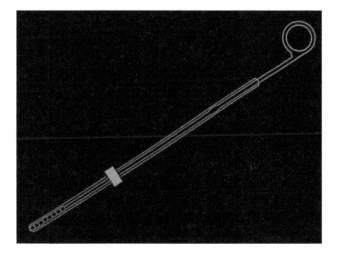

Figure 11.7 Quinacrine tablet inserter.

minilaparotomy include those of the anesthetic, immediate surgical complications (trauma, hemorrhage), and delayed problems (hemorrhage, infection, and failure).

In resource-scarce settings, there is an urgent need for a non-surgical, transcervical method of tubal blockage. In the 1970s, Jaime Zipper in Chile (who had so advanced IUD technology by adding copper to plastic devices) used a small inserter (about the size of a drinking straw) to place pellets of quinacrine in the uterus (Figure 11.7). These dissolve and

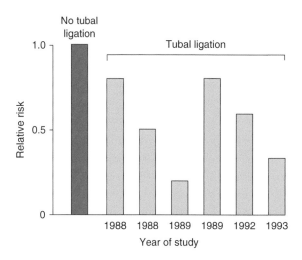

Figure 11.8 Relative risk of ovarian cancer after tubal ligation. (From reference 1 with permission.)

destroy the endometrium and the cells lining the Fallopian tubes. The endometrium regenerates after this 'chemical curettage', but the tubes become fibrosed. The method is simpler than having an IUD inserted: it does have a failure rate and must be repeated at least once. Among 32 000 quinacrine procedures in Vietnam, there were no recorded deaths, whereas over 200 maternal deaths would have occurred in this group of women without sterilization. Studies in several mammalian species using many times the human dose have proved safe, although inflammation and tumor formation occur in rats at 15 times the human dose. Unfortunately, development of the method has become so highly politicized that difficult-to-evaluate data of this sort are unlikely to be evaluated objectively.

Tubal ligation by any route significantly reduces the risk of ovarian cancer, as illustrated in Figure 11.8.

Voluntary surgical contraception should be accepted only when a couple are clear that they want no more children. If disaster strikes, however, and children die prematurely or divorce occurs, then techniques for attempting to restore fertility exist. In the female they involve major operative surgery and, even when successful, carry an inevitable risk of a tubal instead of a uterine pregnancy. In the male, reversal is somewhat easier and does not carry any comparable risk; however, although patency of tubes can be achieved, fertility cannot always be guaranteed.

THE POSSIBILITY OF REGRET

A number of studies have been carried out on the possible long-term sequelae of voluntary sterilization. Regret is more common when the decision to operate is made after an abortion than at an emotionally less charged time.

In some ways many people may regret the end of childbearing, but like wrong false teeth, it may still be the best decision the circumstances permit. In a follow-up of women having tubal ligations in Latin America, as many women regretted not having the operation earlier in their lives as felt they had chosen the operation too soon.

REFERENCE

1. Hankinson SE, Hunter DJ, Colditz GA et al. Tubal ligation, hysterectomy, and risk of ovarian cancer. JAMA 1993; 270: 2813–18.

CHAPTER 12

Contraception for special groups

All currently available methods of modern contraceptives are safe, effective, and reliable. As such, they are suitable for most individuals. However, contraceptive needs differ for different groups of individuals, and also within groups. For example, the contraceptive needs of the young unmarried girl will be different to those of a young married couple in a stable union. Again, the needs of the couple will vary, depending on whether they are delaying the first pregnancy or whether they need a method to space between pregnancies. The same couple's needs will change once their family is complete, when they would do better with a more permanent method. Just as contraceptive needs differ at different stages of one's reproductive life, similarly, specific groups of individuals can be identified who may have specific contraceptive needs. Although there are many such groups, a few important groups will be highlighted.

ADOLESCENTS

Scientific basis for adolescents' behavior

High-powered magnetic resonance imaging (MRI) has made it possible for scientists to study the development of the living human brain. A child's brain is 90–95% of the adult size by the age of 6 years. We are born equipped with most of the neurons our brain will ever have, and in the past it was thought that the brain was largely a finished product by the time a child reached the age of 12 years. Some theorists concluded that the idea of adolescence was an artificial construct, invented in the post-Industrial Revolution years. MRI studies by Giedd[1] in California and elsewhere showed what every parent of a teenager knows: the brain of an adolescent is far from mature, yet often predisposed to risk-taking. The wild conduct once blamed on 'raging hormones' is being seen as the by-product of two factors: a surfeit of sex hormones combined with a paucity of cognitive controls needed for mature behavior.

Between the 3rd and 6th month of gestation, there is an explosive period of prenatal neural growth. What Giedd's long-term studies have shown is that there is a second wave of proliferation and pruning that occurs later in childhood, and that the final critical path of this second wave, affecting some of the highest mental functions, occurs in the late teens.

No matter how a particular brain turns out, its development proceeds in stages, generally from back to front. Some of the brain regions that reach maturity earliest – through proliferation and pruning – are those in the back of the brain that mediate direct contact with the environment by controlling such sensory functions as vision, hearing, touch, and spatial processing. Next are areas that help to coordinate those functions. The very last part of the brain to be pruned and shaped is the prefrontal cortex, home of the so-called executive functions – planning, setting priorities, organizing thoughts, suppressing impulses, and weighing the consequences of one's actions. In other words, the final part of the brain to develop is the part capable of decision-making.

However, hormones remain an important part of the teen brain story. Right about the time the brain switches from proliferating to pruning, the body comes under the hormonal assault of puberty. Hormones released from the ovaries, testes, and adrenal glands act on the brain's emotional center, the limbic system. This creates a 'tinderbox of emotions' says Dr Ronald Dahl, a psychiatrist at the University of Pittsburgh. Not only do feelings reach a flash point more easily but also adolescents tend to seek out situations where they can allow their emotions and passions to run wild: 'It is a very important hint that there is some particular hormone–brain relationship contributing to the appetite for thrills, strong sensations and excitement'. This thrill-seeking may have evolved to promote exploration, an eagerness to leave the nest, and to seek one's own path and partner. But in a world where fast cars, illicit drugs, gangs, and dangerous liaisons beckon, it also puts the teenager at risk.

That is especially so because the brain regions that put the brakes on risky impulsive behavior are still under construction.

Global situation

More than 1 billion girls and boys around the world are in their second decade of life. About 85% of these young people live in developing countries. (The World Health Organization [WHO] defines adolescents as between 10 and 19 years of age and 'young people' as between the ages of 10 and 24.) Young people face enormous challenges to learn, form relationships, shape their identities, and acquire the social and practical skills they need to become active and productive adults. Adults, parents, decision-makers, and the world community at large have a moral and legal obligation to ensure the rights of adolescents, and help them develop their strengths in a supportive and safe environment.

The rights of young people have been affirmed in The Convention on the Rights of the Child Article 2, adopted and opened for signature, ratification, and accession by General Assembly resolution 44/25 of 20 November 1989, Office of the United Nations High Commissioner for Human Rights, Geneva, Switzerland.[2]

All young people have the right to:

- Policies and programs that promote their survival and personal development, including health care, education, life and livelihood skills, and vocational training.
- The highest attainable standard of physical and mental health.
- Protection against violence, discrimination and exploitation.
- Participate in matters that affect their lives and freely express their viewpoints.

These rights have been set out in:

- The Convention on the Rights of the Child.[2]
- The Convention on the Elimination of all Forms of Discrimination against Women, adopted by the United Nations General Assembly in 1979.[3]
- The Programme of Action adopted at the International Conference on Population and Development (ICPD) in 1994[4] and in the key outcome document issued at ICPD+5 in 1999.
- The Beijing Declaration and Platform for Action, adopted at the Fourth World Conference on Women 1995, and the Political Declaration and the outcome document from Beijing +5 in 2000.
- Millennium Development Goals (MDGs) and young people.

The MDGs emanating from the Millennium Summit of the United Nations form a framework for the UN system to work together with governments, non-governmental organizations (NGOs), private sector, and all others concerned to achieve these goals.[5] A number of issues affecting adolescents is central to the MDGs: completion of primary schooling; elimination of gender disparity in primary and secondary education; halting the spread of HIV/AIDS; reducing the maternal mortality ratio; and implementing strategies for decent and productive work for youth. At the country level, the MDGs are supplemented by other development frameworks such as poverty reduction strategies, sector-wide approaches, and health sector reforms.

Many parts of the world, including the USA, have a long way to go before the sexual and reproductive health needs of their young people are met adequately. Very high pregnancy rates among married and unmarried women under 20 years of age are found in countries all over the world, both developing and developed (Figure 12.1).

These high pregnancy rates constitute a major risk for the health and social well-being of the younger woman and her child (see Chapter 2, Health Rationale section). It is, therefore, important to protect the young woman from pregnancy by ensuring contraceptives are accessible to those who need them, and recognizing that, however well contraceptives are used, there will always be some young women who need access to safe abortions. In the USA, for example, over half of the 1.3 million induced abortions per year are obtained by women below age 25, about 33% in teenagers with the rate peaking at ages 18–19 years old.

In almost all countries of the world, the age of puberty is decreasing (Chapter 2) and yet girls are marrying later. Although physically mature, they are not considered socially mature and ready for marriage. This gap has been termed the 'biosocial gap' and it is widening (Figure 12.2). In many countries the age of first intercourse is also falling. These factors result in increasing numbers of pregnancies in unmarried adolescents.[8] In other more traditional societies girls still marry at a young age.

For young women there are some specific hazards associated with early sexuality. For example, the tissues of the cervical epithelium seem more susceptible to dysplasia under the precipitating influence of one or several factors contributed to by the male. Relationships tend to be less stable, and if there is more than one partner involved, there will be the increased risk of sexually transmissible infections and pelvic inflammatory disease. These in turn can lead to sterility or an increased risk of ectopic pregnancy. However, the birth of children to inexperienced and immature mothers is possibly the most complex in its consequences. This situation is made worse when there is inadequate social support.

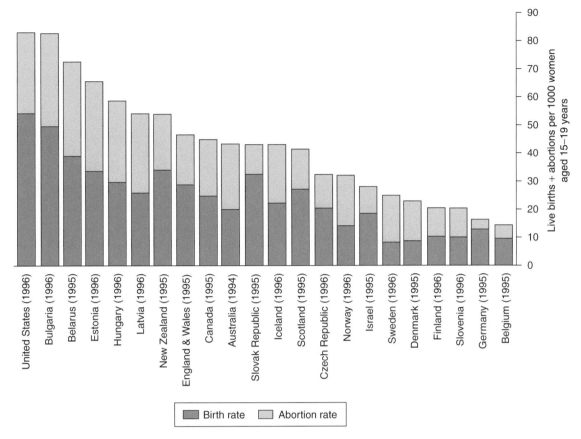

Figure 12.1 International comparisons of teenage pregnancy rates, 2001. Note: these rates do not include fetal loss; pregnancies are calculated here as the sum of live births and abortions. Based on data from the Alan Guttmacher Institute, an independent, not-for-profit organization in the USA, whose mandate is to inform individual decision-making, encourage scientific inquiry, and enlightened public debate, and promote the formation of sound public and private sector programs and policies, related to sexual behavior, reproduction, and family formation. (Reproduced from reference 6, with permission.)

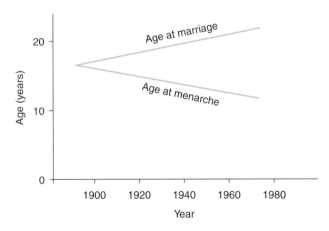

Figure 12.2 The 'biosocial gap' – the gap between age at marriage and age at menarche, 1900–1980. (From reference 7, with permission.)

Reproductive health clinics serving young people should provide an attractive and informal setting, staffed by well-trained and caring people who are not likely to prejudge the moral issues or adversely stereotype their clients. Ideally, counseling should be available for young people of either sex.

No single method of contraception can be considered suitable for adolescents as a group, but factors such as age, parity, sexual habits, risk of infection, risk of pregnancy, the need to conceal the sexual activity, and contraceptive use, should be considered prior to providing a method. The combined oral contraceptive is the most popular and most requested method of contraception by teenagers. This is appropriate because oral contraceptives are almost never medically contraindicated in healthy adolescents. Added advantages for them would be improvement of acne, reduction of menstrual flow and dysmenorrhea, and reduced risk of pelvic inflammatory disease.

Other hormonal methods such as injectables and implants can be used in older adolescents. Although their long-acting feature improves the continuity of use of these methods, there are concerns about depletion of bone density with depot medroxyprogesterone acetate, which may result in adolescents not achieving their peak bone mineral density.

Intrauterine devices (IUDs) are not the method of first choice for nulliparous women or a woman who is likely to have more than one partner.

Barrier methods, including diaphragms and condoms (male and female), are good methods of contraception for highly motivated adolescents who are able to use these methods consistently and correctly, mainly because adolescents change their partners more frequently and are at a higher risk of sexually transmitted infections, including HIV.

Spermicides, when used with diaphragms or condoms, ensure high effectiveness. Used alone, they are less effective; but they are usually easy to obtain and use, and this may be an advantage, particularly for adolescents. Withdrawal and periodic abstinence are not reliable methods, particularly for the adolescent. In adolescents, sexual control may be low, leading to higher failure rates with coitus interruptus. Periodic abstinence relies on attempts to identify the time of ovulation and this is dependent on regular cycles, which may not occur in the early reproductive years. This method is also difficult to use by those who only have occasional sexual intercourse.

Sterilization is rarely indicated in this age group and should be considered only in exceptional medically dictated circumstances where a pregnancy would pose a life-threatening risk to the mother.

It is essential that adolescents should be made aware of emergency contraceptive methods, although they should be advised not to use them as a regular solution to unprotected intercourse.

CONTRACEPTION FOR THE OLDER WOMAN

For women over 35 years of age (regarded obstetrically as 'older women') there are particular needs and problems associated with contraception. The ability to conceive continues to decrease with age until the menopause. So these women, on the one hand, may not need very effective methods of contraception. However, on the other hand, an accidental pregnancy for a woman in her forties carries an increased risk for fetal chromosomal anomalies; spontaneous abortions; antenatal, intrapartum, and postpartum complications; and maternal morbidity and mortality. So a balance has to be struck. Women in this age group may be more prone to conditions such as obesity, hypertension, and diabetes which, together with smoking, are risk factors for adverse cardiovascular effects when taking oral contraceptives. Figure 12.3 illustrates the relationship between estrogen and progesterone dosage of combined oral contraceptives and the incidence of total arterial disease. At the lowest dosage of estrogen and progesterone, no deaths were seen. However, at

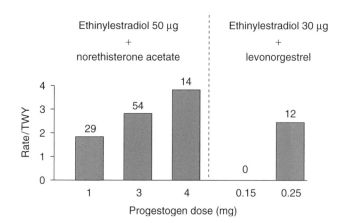

Figure 12.3 Incidence of arterial diseases during oral contraceptive use per 1000 woman-years (TWY). (From reference 9, with permission.)

the same time, these women should also be made aware of the non-contraceptive benefits of hormonal contraception (see Figure 6.2).

Sterilization is a suitable option for many women over 35 years old, and female sterilization or vasectomy is being selected increasingly by couples of this age group whose family size is complete. Both procedures have very low rates of failure and the simple operation can be carried out under local anesthetic.

Combined oral contraceptives can be used for the older woman who has minimal risk factors for cardiovascular complications. Even women over 40 years old who have no risk factors can still consider using the combined pill with appropriate information. The progestogen-only pill, on the other hand, is suitable for women until menopause.

Other hormonal methods such as injectables or implants can be useful for the older woman. However, injectables are believed to cause an increase in blood pressure in susceptible older women, and long-term use is not recommended. The IUD is another method suitable for older women. Menstrual loss can be increased and women should be warned, particularly at this age, about this side effect. Where other symptoms of menopause exist, devices should be removed about 1 year before menopause. This will enable the woman to know if the bleeding she has is due to the device or due to menstruation. On the other hand, there are advantages of removing the IUD after menopause.

The protection IUDs offer can be long term. In the absence of complications, copper devices may be left in for 10 years or more. Those inserted after age 40 years may be left in until menopause, unless a woman becomes pregnant. An IUD should be removed 1 year after menses stop, but no ill effects have been reported among women who have not had them removed more than 1 year after menopause.[10]

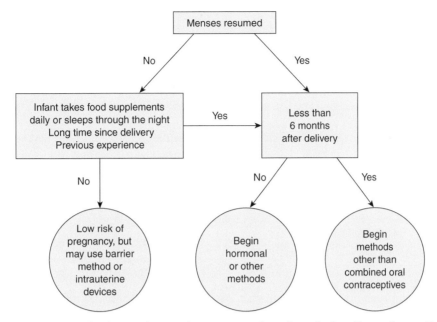

Figure 12.4 A simplified decision tree for the introduction of contraception during breastfeeding. (From reference 7, with permission.)

Barrier methods are often acceptable to older women, and may be suitable, particularly since fertility at this age is reduced and pregnancy rates are low.

CONTRACEPTION FOR NURSING MOTHERS

The choice of method of contraception for breastfeeding mothers is important because the chosen methods, in addition to providing effective contraception, must not adversely affect the quantity and quality of breast milk or the health of the infant. The method, and when to start the method, are both important considerations.

There are no universal rules in determining when a breastfeeding woman should start a particular contraceptive method. The best solution may be the formation of a decision tree adapted to a woman's specific situation. An example of this is shown in Figure 12.4.

Over the past few years a consensus has developed among medical professionals and family planning experts that breastfeeding, under the right conditions, can be used as a reliable contraceptive. Briefly, the conditions for the lactational amenorrhea method (LAM) are as follows:

- the mother has not experienced vaginal bleeding after the 8 weeks' postpartum
- the baby is less than 6 months old
- the baby receives all of its nutrition from the breast, without bottles, supplements, or solid food

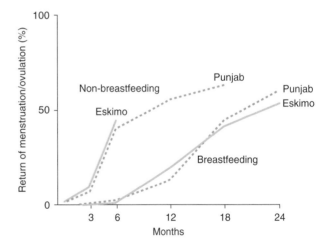

Figure 12.5 Return of menstruation/ovulation in bottle-feeding mothers and breastfeeding mothers.

- the baby feeds at the breast at least every 4 hours during the day and every 6 hours at night.

A woman who meets the above criteria has a greater than 98% chance of not becoming pregnant, which compares well with other forms of contraception.

In countries where the duration of breastfeeding is long (e.g. median duration in Senegal 19 months, in Bangladesh 31 months) breastfeeding contributes greatly to delaying conception. It is important to remember that the effect of breastfeeding on fertility is significant primarily during the period before menses return (Figures 12.5 and 12.6).

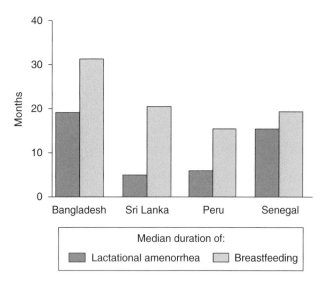

Figure 12.6 Duration of breastfeeding and lactational amenorrhea. (From references 11 and 12.)

Breastfeeding: does it really space babies?

A professor of pediatrics put it this way:

> Demographic data recorded prior to the 20th century from birth records all over the world indicate that the average spacing of children was about two years when mother's milk supplied the major source of calories for infants during the first year to 1.5 years of life.[13]

This was confirmed by a conference on lactation infertility (Bellagio, Italy, 1988), which stated:

> Demographic data indicate that in many developing countries, the protection from pregnancy provided by breastfeeding alone is greater than that given by all other reversible means of family planning combined ... Postpartum women should be offered a choice of using breastfeeding as a means of family planning, either to help achieve optimal birth spacing of two years, or as a way of delaying the introduction of other contraceptives.[14]

Furthermore, it is now recognized that it is not just any kind of breastfeeding that spaces babies. That's why the Bellagio conference added: 'They (the mothers) should be informed how to maximize the antifertility effects of breastfeeding to prevent pregnancy.' What that means is this: only 'ecological' breastfeeding provides extended postpartum infertility. This is a form of baby care which is characterized by constant mother–baby togetherness and frequent nursing, both by day and by night.

On the average, however, true ecological breastfeeding will space babies about 2 years apart, even in North American culture.

The key to breastfeeding infertility is frequent suckling and that is simply a part of natural mothering which entails mother–baby inseparability. When mother goes to church, so does baby. When mother goes shopping, attends a meeting, or visits a friend, so does baby. And when baby indicates a need to nurse, mother obliges. When mother goes to bed at night, baby is either in the same bed, or at least the child's bed is right next to the parents' bed so that baby can nurse off and on during the night without any fuss and bother.

Eventually fertility returns. Usually, but not always, it is preceded by a 'warning menstrual period' and frequently the first menstrual cycle will be infertile (sometimes others as well).

While the chances of pregnancy are at the 1% level during the first 6 months postpartum prior to the first menstruation, after 6 months the chance of pregnancy increases. Three studies have indicated that the actual rate of pregnancy is about 6%, a rate that is very competitive with actual use rates for both natural and artifical methods of birth control.

Conclusions

Breastfeeding is best for both mothers and babies and should be encouraged. Breastfeeding can also provide natural, safe, effective contraceptive protection, if certain conditions are met, for up to 6 months postpartum. Women who are interested in using the natural protection of breastfeeding should have access to information about LAM and about other available family planning methods suitable for breastfeeding women.[15]

Compared with other contraceptive methods such as the condom and even the oral contraceptive pill, the LAM can be highly effective in preventing pregnancy if used in the typical manner (Table 12.1). If the mother decides to breastfeed, then she should be supported to carry out the decision. Support, for example, in the form of good nutrition, maternity leave, and assistance on how to breastfeed should be made available. The option for these mothers to rely on the contraceptive effects of lactation should be carefully explained. Provided the mother understands and accepts the possibility of an unexpected early conception (2% of mothers

Table 12.1 Pregnancy rates per 100 women using lactational amenorrhea method (LAM), compared with standard methods of contraception, in the first 12 months of use

	Typical use	Perfect use
Injectables	0.3	0.3
IUD	0.8	0.6
LAM	2	0.5
Combined oral contraceptives	6–8	0.1
Condom	14	3

From reference 16, with permission.

Table 12.2 Advantages and disadvantages of lactational amenorrhea method

Advantages	Disadvantages
• Very effective • Provides up to 0.5 couple years protection • Has no side effects • Does not require insertion of any device at the time of sexual intercourse • May attract new family planning users • Contributes to family planning prevalence directly and through increased acceptance rates • Can be initiated immediately postpartum • Is economical and requires no commodities or supplies • Contributes to optimal breastfeeding practices and therefore enhances maternal and infant health and nutrition • Acceptable to all religious groups	• Can only be used for a short period (up to 6 months' postpartum) • Requires breastfeeding frequently both day and night

will conceive before menses has resumed and if they are feeding on demand), some of them will find it convenient to breastfeed without the risks and inconvenience of another method of contraception, especially since there are many added advantages of LAM (Table 12.2). Most methods of contraception can be used during lactation, but particular attention is required in relation to hormonal methods.

Combined estrogen–progestogen pills reduce milk volume as well as the duration of lactation and are best avoided, especially during early lactation. If it is necessary to use a combined pill, it is best to use as low a dose as possible, and only after breastfeeding is well established.

If a hormonal method is to be used during lactation, progestogen-only preparations have the advantage that they appear to have little or no adverse effects on milk production (quality and volume). Injectables, implants containing only progestogens can also be used. There is also much to be said in favor of non-hormonal methods for breastfeeding mothers and IUDs, barrier methods, and spermicides can also be used effectively during lactation.

Postpartum female sterilization is a simple procedure and is commonly performed under local anesthesia. If sterilization is performed immediately after delivery, there is no effect on milk output, but if the operation is carried out after 7–14 days, the procedure is associated with a sharp drop in milk volume. Alternatively, sterilization can be delayed until 6 weeks' postpartum when the uterus has involuted and laparoscopic or minilaparotomy sterilization can be performed. Counseling is important prior to providing any method of contraception. In particular, adequate counseling is vital when postpartum procedures are carried out since the mother may not be in a state of mind to give full informed consent, and also because her decision may have to be based following full assessment of the health status of the newborn infant.

CONTRACEPTION FOR PERSONS WITH DISABILITIES

Attitudes towards the personal and sexual needs of the disabled are changing, not least among the disabled themselves. Most disabled people want to lead as normal a life as possible and that may mean getting married and having children.

If the physical disability affects sexual function, particularly for men who may not be able to sustain an erection and/or who may be infertile (for example, in spinal cord injury, spina bifida, and advanced stages of multiple sclerosis), then contraception is not an issue. However, many women suffering from some disorders are able to become pregnant. The choice of contraceptive will have to be decided by considering primarily the woman's needs with regard to whether she wants to get pregnant or not.

If she wants to postpone pregnancy or not get pregnant at all, the choice of method would once again depend very much on her disability, her partner's support, and also on the type of method that she could use on a continuing basis.

At the beginning of the 20th century, mentally handicapped females were subjected to compulsory sterilization, with the aim of preventing the propagation of this disability in future generations. Hysterectomies performed early in such individuals served multiple purposes, including eliminating the need for further gynecological care. However, more recently, the rights of the mentally handicapped have been recognized, and a number of laws have been introduced to ensure the protection of these rights. Many such laws prohibit sterilization unless an ethical review committee can decide whether the procedure should or should not be done.

Although details of specific methods of contraception for the disabled cannot be prescribed in a general fashion in a book such as this, it suffices to alert the reader to the fact that the disabled person has rights similar to those enjoyed by 'normal' individuals and those caring for the disabled should consider the sexuality of the disabled with regard to the provision of health care and family planning services.

CONTRACEPTION IN WOMEN WITH SERIOUS MEDICAL ILLNESSES

Over 10% of women of reproductive age will have experienced a serious chronic physical disorder, of which the most prevalent disorders are heart disease, hypertension, diabetes mellitus, and renal disease. Ideally, family planning should be an intrinsic part of the total care of such a woman, yet reproductive health issues, including contraception, are all too often ignored.

While medical disorders complicate pregnancy, pregnancy itself aggravates medical disorders. In certain medical disorders, pregnancy is contraindicated due to its endangering effects on the life of the mother. Medical disorders complicating pregnancy account for a significant number of maternal deaths the world over, even though obstetric care has improved over the years. Therefore, the knowledge and practice of contraception plays a major role in preventing maternal and fetal deaths in these women.

In women with cardiac disease, both the cardiovascular sequelae of pregnancy should the contraceptive fail, and the potential adverse circulatory effects of various contraceptive methods, must be considered. In women with hypertension, increased risk of arterial thrombosis associated with the combined pill should be taken into consideration. Along with hypertension, obese women who smoke run a greater risk for thromboembolism. Although glycemic control may be difficult when using combined oral pills in women with diabetes, the real concern is aggravation of vascular disease associated with diabetes. In women with neurological disease, a method must be selected that will not interact with anticonvulsants or immunosuppressive medications. In addition, the indications and contraindications of contraceptive methods for women with pulmonary, gastrointestinal, endocrine, hematological, renal, and rheumatological disease; HIV/AIDS; cancer; and psychiatric morbidity should be closely discussed and considered. Table 12.3 reviews World Health Organization medical eligibility criteria for use of the major contraceptive methods.

Women with conditions that may make pregnancy an unacceptable health risk should be counseled about the higher chances they face with regards to typical-use failure rates. Therefore, the sole use of barrier methods for contraception and behavior-based methods of contraception may not be the most suitable option for them and voluntary sterilization can be a sensible choice. Some of these medical conditions are listed in Table 12.3.

CONTRACEPTION IN SITUATIONS OF HUMANITARIAN CRISES

From time to time, human beings are thrust into precarious and vulnerable situations over which they have no control, during which the lives of entire communities are uncompromisingly threatened. Natural disasters, wars, and armed conflicts have a tendency to strike when mankind is least prepared, and in their wake bring about many new problems which could affect those involved for generations to come. In December 2004, the tsunami disaster, which devastated many countries in East Asia, killing more than 280 000 people and displacing millions, created a collapse of the health systems in many countries.

Crises such as the above disrupt the health system, and thus render access to contraception and other health services difficult, and often impossible. The implications of such a situation can be even more disastrous than the calamity itself. Women and children in particular are exposed to unfortunate incidences of rape, unintended pregnancies, unsafe abortions, spread of HIV and other sexually transmitted diseases, as well as the long-term psychological sequelae of such, and effects on infant and maternal mortality. Out of the 35 million internally displaced refugees in the world today, 80% are women and children.[19] Amidst the chaos of the tsunami, an increasing number of rapes were reported in countries such as Sri Lanka and Indonesia.[19] During the genocide in Rwanda, an estimated half a million females were raped, out of which 67% contracted the HIV virus, thus actually triggering the country's HIV/AIDS epidemic.[18]

The death of the family breadwinner, or the destruction of a family's means of income, may force those women and children left behind into 'survival sex'. Displacement of the defenseless into refugee camps may actually increase their risk of being sexually violated. The mental turmoil of a natural disaster may push people towards entering into casual sexual relationships as a means of emotional support. Overcrowding within refugee camps, and the arrival of military, relief, and reconstruction personnel may lead to promiscuity or forced sexual encounters with the resultant spread of sexually transmitted diseases. All these factors are important to consider in light of the fact that contraceptive supplies are also lost, and often take many weeks for stocks to be replenished. It has often been observed in humanitarian crises that the priority given for providing early distribution of contraceptives is quite low. A month after the tsunami, Indonesia had to appeal to international aid providers regarding their increasingly unmet need for contraception.

The fundamental obligation to safeguard the reproductive health of communities during a humanitarian crisis has been

Table 12.3 WHO medical eligibility criteria for the use of major contraceptive methods

	COCs	POCs	DMPA/NETEN	NP	FS	Vas	Condoms	IUD	Spermicides	Dia/CC	FAMB	LAM
Pregnant	N/A	N/A	N/A	N/A	Delay	—	—	4	—	—	—	—
Age												
<18 years old (<20 years old for IUD)	1	1	2	1	Caution[3]	—[a]	—	2	—	—	—[b,c]	—
18–39 years old	1	1	1	1	Accept[a]	—[a]	—	1	—	—	—	—
40–45 years old	2	1	1	1	Accept[a]	—[a]	—	1	—	—	—[b,c]	—
>45 years old	2	1	2	1	Accept[a]	—[a]	—	1	—	—	—[b,c]	—
Smoking												
<35 years old	2	1	1	1	Accept[a]	—[a]	—	1	—	—	—	—
≥35 years old												
Light smoker (fewer than 15 cigarettes/day)	3	1	1	1	Accept[a]	—[a]	—	1	—	—	—	—
Heavy smoker (≥15 cigarettes/day)	4	1	1	1	Accept[a]	—[a]	—	1	—	—	—	—
High blood pressure (hypertension)												
Systolic 140–159 or diastolic 90–99 mmHg	3	1	2	1	Caution	—	—	1	—	—	—	—[d]
Systolic 160 mmHg and over or diastolic ≥100 mmHg	4	2	3	2	Refer	—	—[d]	1	—[d]	—[d]	—[d]	—
Adequately controlled hypertension where blood pressure can be monitored	3	1	2	1	Caution	—	—	1	—	—	—	—[d]
Past hypertension where blood pressure cannot be evaluated	3	2	2	2	Caution	—	—	1	—	—	—	—
Diabetes												
Past elevated blood sugar levels during pregnancy	1	1	1	1	Accept	—	—	1	—	—	—	—
Diabetes without vascular disease												

COCs, combined oral contraceptives; POCs, progestin-only oral contraceptives; DMPA/NETEN, NP, Norplant implants; FS, female sterilization; Vas, vasectomy; IUD, TCu-380A intrauterine device; Dia/CC, diaphragm/cervical cap, FABM, fertility awareness-based methods, LAM, lactational amenorrhea method.

N/A, not applicable to decision to use method.

—, Condition not listed by WHO for this method; does not affect eligibility for method use.

[a] Sterilization is appropriate for women and men of any age, but only if they are sure they will not want children in the future.

[b] This condition may affect ovarian function and/or change fertility signs and symptoms and/or make methods difficult to learn and use.

[c] Shortly after menarche (age at first menstrual bleeding) and as menopause approaches, menstrual cycles may be irregular.

[d] Breastfeeding may not be recommended with drugs used to treat this condition.

From reference 17.

Table 12.4 Conditions that expose a woman to increased risk as a result of unintended pregnancy

Breast cancer
Complicated valvular heart disease
Diabetes: insulin-dependent; with nephropathy/retinopathy/neuropathy or other vascular disease; or of >20 years' duration
Endometrial or ovarian cancer
High blood pressure (systolic >160 mmHg or diastolic >100 mmHg)[a]
HIV/AIDS[b]
Ischemic heart disease
Malignant gestational trophoblastic disease
Malignant liver tumors (hepatoma)
Schistosomiasis with fibrosis of the liver
Severe (decompensated) cirrhosis
Sickle cell disease
Sexually transmitted infection[b]
Stroke
Thrombogenic mutations
Tuberculosis

[a]Throughout this atlas, blood pressure measurements are given in mmHg. To convert to kPa, multiply by 0.1333. For example, 120/80 mmHg = 16.0/10.7 kPa.
[b]Dual protection is strongly recommended for protection against HIV/AIDS and other sexually transmitted infections (STIs) when a risk of STI/HIV transmission exists. This can be achieved through the simultaneous use of condoms with other methods or the consistent and correct use of condoms alone.

increasingly appreciated by international organizations. In 1995, a coalition between UN agencies, governments, and NGOs resulted in the establishment of the International Agency Working Group on Reproductive Health in Refugee Situations.[18] Their work involved the creation of an Emergency Reproductive Health Kit, which consists of critical requirements during such emergency situations, such as male and female condoms, rape treatment health supplies, oral and injectable contraception, IUDs, treatment for sexually transmitted infections, and equipment for clean delivery. These kits have been successfully used in countries such as Bosnia, Macedonia, Albania, Sierra Leone, Congo, and Liberia during disaster situations, and were also of much value during the recent tsunami crisis.[19]

Other similar services, which have been set up by international aid agencies, are the Minimal Initial Service Package (MISP), a concept of the Interagency Symposium on Reproductive Health in Emergency Situations in 1995, which mainly focuses on preventing and managing consequences of sexual violence, reducing transmission of HIV through universal precautions and condoms, and facilitating safe deliveries.[19]

The UNFPA has also helped many countries during catastrophes, such as Sierra Leone and Guinea, by organizing massive awareness-raising campaigns for refugees regarding HIV, sexually transmitted infections, and prevention of unintended pregnancies. They have also provided free male and female condoms as a first line of defense.[14]

Emergency contraception in crisis situations

Most women who have been exposed to an unprotected sexual encounter, either voluntarily or by force, are not even aware that something can be done to prevent pregnancy. This is especially the case in crisis situations, where, with all the tumult and struggle for the basic necessities of life, the fear of pregnancy is probably the last thing that occurs in their minds. Furthermore, most victims of rape are unwilling to report the assault due to shame or fear of being blamed, and therefore unwilling to seek services. Health care workers should pay particular attention to the above issues in situations of a crisis. Emergency healthcare centers and other relief operations should be equipped with the means for emergency contraception when and where it is required.

The emergency contraceptive pills have much value in such situations. There are two currently popular regimens of hormonal preparations that can be used: the levonorgestrel-only regimen and the combined estrogen–progestin (Yuzpe) regimen (see Chapter 6). The latter is associated with an increased incidence of nausea and vomiting, and therefore should be reserved for situations where the former is unavailable.

Another method of emergency contraception that can be used is the copper-bearing IUD (see Chapter 9). It has the added benefit that it can be left in place for women who require long-term contraception, or are at continuous risk of being further sexually victimized. It can also be inserted up to 5 days after the unprotected exposure, and therefore may provide protection to women in areas where health service provision has been somewhat delayed. However, trained personnel are required for the processes of insertion as well as screening clients for suitability. If sexually transmitted infections are rampant within a refugee camp, it may be unwise to opt for IUDs as a method of emergency contraception.[20]

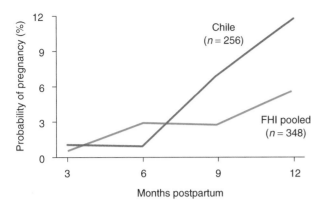

Figure 12.7 Cumulative probability of pregnancy during lactational amenorrhea. FHI.

Reversing sterilization

During the aftermath of the tsunami, an important issue that surfaced was the increasing number of requests for reversal of sterilization. In Tamil Nadu, 2300 children under the age of 18 died during the tsunami, and by that time, 44% of women who had already borne two children had been sterilized.[19]

Reversal of sterilization may not always be successful despite the fact that modern surgical techniques have rendered the process quite simple (see Chapter 11). When a couple embarks on the decision for sterilization, they certainly do not expect to request its reversal one day in the future. However, with the increasing number of man-made and natural calamities that affect us today, perhaps we should think twice about the role sterilization should actually play in family planning, when easily reversible, yet perhaps equally effective methods such as IUDs and hormonal implants exist as possible options for most of these women.

Abortion

Access to safe abortion is essential, especially for women who have been raped, and health workers need to be sensitive to the fact that many women are reluctant to report rape.

REFERENCES

1. Giedd JN. Adolescent brain development: vulnerabilities and opportunities. Ann NY Acad Sci 2004; 1021: 77–85.
2. The Convention on the Rights of the Child, 1989. Geneva, Switzerland: Office of the UN High Commissioner of Human Rights.
3. The Convention on the Elimination of all Forms of Discrimination against Women, 1979. New York: UN General Assembly, 1979. http://en.wikipedia.org/wiki/convention on the elimination of all forms of discrimination against women
4. The Programme of Action. International Conference on Population and Development, September 1994.
5. Millennium Development Goals. Kofi Annan, Secretary General of United Nations. New York: UN Department of Public Information, 2000.
6. Darroch JE, Singh S, Frost JJ et al. Differences in teenage pregnancy rates among five developed countries: the roles of sexual activity and contraceptive use. Family Planning Perspectives 2001; 33: 246.
7. Rosenfield A, Fathalla MD. The FIGO Manual of Human Reproduction. Carnforth, UK: Parthenon, 1990.
8. A Clinical Guide for CP, 4th edn. 2005: 329.
9. Kay CR. The Royal College of General Practitioners' Oral Contraception Study: some recent observations. Clin Obstet Gynaecol 1984; 11: 759–86.
10. Family Health International Network 1996; 16(2).
11. World Fertility Survey, Bangladesh, 1979.
12. Demographic and Health Surveys, Peru, 1986; Senegal, 1986; Sri Lanka, 1987.
13. Jackson RL. Ecological breastfeeding and child spacing. Clin Pediatr (Phila) 1988; 27(8): 373–7.
14. Kennedy KI, Rivera R, McNeilly AS. Consensus statement on the use of breastfeeding as a family planning method. Contraception 1989; 39(5): 477–96.
15. Labbok M, Cooney K, Coly S. Guidelines: Breastfeeding, Family Planning and the Lactational Amenorrhea Method – LAM. Washington, DC: Institute for Reproductive Health, 1994.
16. Essentials of Contraceptive Technology. Johns Hopkins Population Information Program, 1997.
17. World Health Organization. Improving Access to Quality Care in Family Planning Sevices: Medical Eligibility Criteria for Contraceptive Use, 2nd ed. 2002.
18. Heyzer N. UNFPA State of World Population 2005. Women and young people in humanitarian crises. In: The Promise of Equality: Gender Equity, Reproductive Health, and the Millennium Development Goals 2005: 75–83.
19. Carballo M, Herdandez M, Schneider K, Welle E. Impact of the tsunami on reproductive health. J R Soc Med 2005; 98: 400–3.
20. Expanding global access to emergency contraception. A collaborative approach to meeting women's needs. Consortium for Emergency Contraception, October 2000, Emergency Contraceptive pills: Medical and Service Delivery Guidelines, 2000: 47–48.

CHAPTER 13

Abortion

The Alan Guttmacher Institute in New York estimates that a woman now entering her fertile years will on average have one abortion. Yet abortion is as controversial as it is common. The very term 'abortion' conjures up many opinions – whether it is safe or unsafe, legal or illegal, right or wrong. Not surprisingly, many people are ambivalent about abortion. The outcome of surveys depends on how questions are posed. In 1987 in a secret ballot and by a two to one majority, the citizens of Ireland voted to amend the constitution to protect the 'unborn child', yet when in 1992 a 14-year-old girl was pregnant as a result of rape, two-thirds of the population supported her right to travel to London to obtain an abortion. Moreover, in the real world, many of those who are ambivalent about whether to deny another woman an abortion, may well seek a safe abortion when they – or their wife or daughter – have an unwanted pregnancy.

Much can be learnt from the experience of different countries. No society has ever achieved a small family size without resorting to abortion, whether legal or illegal. Nevertheless, the number of abortions that occur in a society is highly influenced by access to contraception. Statistics from Russia, the USA, and the Netherlands illustrate this point. All have similar birth rates but in Russia contraceptives are difficult to obtain and are of poor quality (for good reasons: in the Russian language 'condoms' are galoshes), and voluntary surgical contraception is not offered. As a result, well over 6 million abortions are registered each year. In addition, many doctors take payment from the woman for a slightly less painful and more private operation, and some estimates put the number of abortions even higher. In the Netherlands contraceptives are widely available and, although abortion is legal, it is a right that is rarely exercised (Figure 13.1). According to the rate per 1000 fertile women, the Netherlands has one-thirtieth of the abortion rate of Russia. The USA has 1.5 million abortions a year, and lies somewhere between Russia and the Netherlands in

its availability of, and attitudes towards, contraception (Table 13.1). Figure 13.2 shows how the problems associated with abortion have decreased as the use of contraceptives has increased.

The majority of the world's population live in countries where abortion is legally available, either on the recommendation of a physician, as in the UK, or at the request of the woman, as in the USA and parts of Eastern Europe. Data comparing abortion rates where the operation is legal or illegal, or where it was illegal and became legal (as in the UK), or the reverse (as in Romania) where it was legal and became illegal, suggest that laws prohibiting abortion do not necessarily reduce the number of abortions taking place, but they do increase the danger to the individual woman immeasurably, as well as creating opportunities for financial and sexual exploitation.

In terms of human suffering and increased mortality, strict antiabortion laws can lead to very counterproductive results. For example, Nicolae Ceauşescu introduced a strict abortion law in Romania in 1966; 9 months later the birth rate doubled. However, an illegal abortion network was established in the country and the birth rate fell back to previous levels, although the maternal mortality rate rose to the highest in Europe (Figure 13.3). Thousands, perhaps tens of thousands of women, died from botched abortions during Ceauşescu's regime. In the year following the death of Ceauşescu and the liberalization of abortion, maternal mortality fell by 55% as unsafe abortions began to disappear.

WHEN DOES LIFE BEGIN?

The problem with abortion is not clinical, but ethical and political. Social surveys show that a minority of people believe that abortion is equivalent to murder and should be outlawed. Another minority group believes that women have an unfettered right over their own reproductive

Africa	
Algeria	Mali
Angola	Mauritania
Benin	Mauritius
Botswana	Morocco
Burkina Faso	Mozambique
Burundi	Namibia
Cameroon	Niger
Cent. Af. Rep.	Nigeria
Chad	Rwanda
Congo	Senegal
Côte d'Ivoire	Sierra Leone
Egypt	Somalia
Ethiopia	South Africa
Gabon	Sudan
Ghana	Tanzania
Guinea	Togo
Kenya	Tunisia
Lesotho	Uganda
Liberia	Zaire
Libya	Zambia
Madagascar	Zimbabwe
Malawi	

Asia & Oceania	
Afghanistan	Malaysia
Australia	Mongolia
Bangladesh	Myanmar (Burma)
Cambodia	Nepal
China	New Zealand
Hong Kong	Oman
India	Pakistan
Indonesia	Papua New Guinea
Iran	Philippines
Iraq	Saudi Arabia
Israel	Singapore
Japan	Sri Lanka
Jordan	Syria
Korea, Dem. Rep.	Taiwan
Korea, Rep. of	Thailand
Kuwait	Turkey
Laos	UAE
Lebanon	Vietnam
	Yemen

The Americas	
Argentina	Haiti
Bolivia	Honduras
Brazil	Jamaica
Canada	Mexico[1]
Chile	Nicaragua
Colombia	Panama
Costa Rica	Paraguay
Cuba	Peru
Dominican Rep.	Puerto Rico
Ecuador	Trinidad & Tob.
El Salvador	United States
Guatemala	Uruguay
Guyana	Venezuela

Europe	
Albania	Ireland
Austria	Italy
Belgium	The Netherlands
Bulgaria	Norway
Czech. Rep.	Northern Ireland
Denmark	Poland
Finland	Portugal
France	Romania
Germany	USSR (former)
Great Britain	Spain
Greece	Sweden
Hungary	Switzerland
Iceland	Yugoslavia (former)

There are four types of abortion laws

Very strict – to save a women's life or under no circumstances

Rather strict – maternal health and/or judicial reasons (rape, incest)

Rather broad – social and social-medical reasons

On request – reasons not specified or on request

Figure 13.1 Abortion laws worldwide. Note, the above classification is intended as a general indicator only, and is not intended to be a precise summary of the legal situation in each country – since details of the law currently in force will differ significantly within the same broad classification band.

[1]This change is limited to Mexico City

Table 13.1 Worldwide incidence of induced abortion

Total number	46 million
Safe abortions	26 million
Unsafe abortions	20 million
Ratio	26/100 pregnancies
Rate	35/1000 women/year
Rate – developing world	34/1000 women/year
Rate – developed world	39/1000 women/year
Lowest rate (the Netherlands)	6.5/1000 women/year
Highest rate (Vietnam)	83.3/1000 women/year

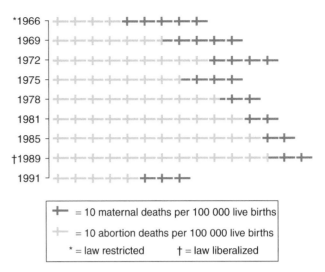

Figure 13.3 Abortion rates and maternal mortality (Romania 1960–1990).

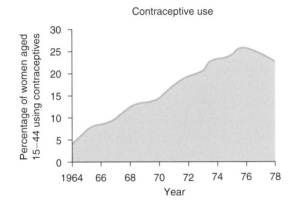

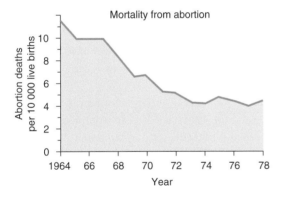

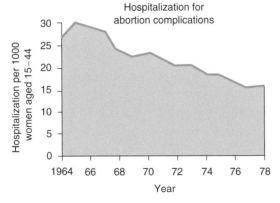

Figure 13.2 Problems from abortion decline as use of contraceptives increases, Chile 1964–78. (From reference 1.)

systems. Most people are uncomfortable with abortion but recognize that, in many cases, it is the most appropriate

solution to the problem. More than 90% of people believe that women ought to be able to have an abortion in cases where the fetus is congenitally abnormal, or the pregnancy follows rape or incest.

Scientifically, embryologists can no more tell when life begins than an astronomer can tell if heaven exists by looking for heaven with a telescope. The ethical and legal status individuals ascribe to the developing embryo is a matter of belief, not observable fact. In the landmark case Roe vs Wade 1972, the US Supreme Court wisely stated:

> We need not resolve the difficult question of when life begins. When those trained in the respective disciplines of medicine, philosophy and theology are unable to arrive at a consensus, the judiciary, at this point in the development of man's knowledge, is not in a position to speculate as to the answer.

In other words, the judgments people make about abortion are based on religious faith and belief.

In any pluralistic society, legislation on abortion should be based on tolerance of a variety of beliefs about life before birth, just as a variety of beliefs about life after death must be accommodated. It should be no more surprising to find an abortion clinic in a city where a significant number of people believe abortion to be murder than it is to find a mosque, a synagogue, and a church – all of which teach different pathways to eternal life – in the same community.

TECHNIQUES OF ABORTION
Safe abortion

In the 19th century, the Scottish obstetrician James Young Simpson described a vacuum technique which he appears to

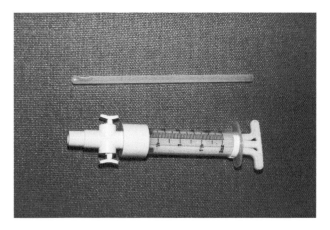

Figure 13.4 Hand-held vacuum syringe and Karman cannula. (Source, International Projects Assistance Services, USA.)

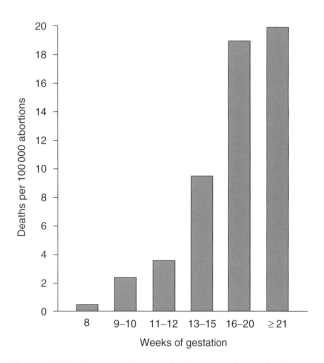

Figure 13.5 Mortality related to legal abortion, by week of gestation, compared with the risk of carrying a pregnancy to term (note that maternal mortality could be as high as 5–600/100 000 live births in some developing countries).

have used to induce early abortions. Working independently and outside the medical profession, Harvey Karman, a California psychologist, developed a flexible plastic cannula with hand-held syringe (Figure 13.4). Manual vaccum aspiration (MVA) is now widely used in many countries and it is a safe, simple way of performing early abortion, whether done under paracervical block or even without any anesthetic at all. Vacuum aspiration is now considered the optimal way of inducing abortion in the first trimester of pregnancy.

Table 13.2 Mortality rate per 100 000 legal abortions, for selected countries before and after access to safe abortion

Country	Mortality rate	Decrease (%)
Canada (1970/75–1976/83)	3.6–0.2	94.0
Czechoslovakia (1975/66–1976/83)	3.8–0.4	89.0
Denmark (1940/50–1976/87)	195–0.7	99.6
England/Wales (1968/69–1980/87)	26–1.3	95.0
Hungary (1957/62–1968/78)	4.1–0.7	83.0
Sweden (1946/48–1980/87)	250–0.4	99.8
USA (1970–1980/85)	19–0.6	97.0

Technically, early abortion is a simple, safe procedure which, when performed with modern techniques, is four or five times as safe as carrying a pregnancy to term. All abortions have greater side effects and risks of death with increasing duration of the pregnancy. Abortion in the first 12 weeks of pregnancy is considered safer than carrying the pregnancy to term. By about the 22nd week of pregnancy, the risks of performing an abortion exceed those of carrying a pregnancy to term (Figure 13.5).

In the first 8 weeks of pregnancy, the uterus can be emptied using a small flexible plastic cannula a little bigger than a drinking straw. Local anesthesia is usually appropriate. After 12 weeks of pregnancy, the operation is clinically more difficult and ethically more challenging. Even so, the long-term follow-up of women who have had abortions has not demonstrated any consistent adverse psychological or physical effects.

With the development of mifepristone (RU-486) in France in the 1980s, medical abortion has become a practical possibility. Mifepristone blocks the action of progesterone. Administered in the first 6 weeks of pregnancy, and followed by the prostaglandin misoprostol (which leads to forceful uterine contractions), abortion can be induced without surgery in over 97% of cases. The woman will experience cramping pains and she may be distressed by the amount of blood lost, but for the first time in history a woman can iduce an abortion safely in her own home.

Unsafe abortions

Every minute, a woman dies in the world from pregnancy, childbirth, or abortion, and in parts of Africa unsafe abortions account for up to one-half of this sad toll. Badly performed abortions are up to 1000 times more dangerous than early vacuum aspiration abortion (Table 13.2). The dangers of abortion are hemorrhage, infection, and perforation of the uterus. In parts of Latin America, botched abortion places the largest single demand on the blood transfusion services. In most months in one hospital in Addis Ababa, Ethiopia, more women die from the consequences of illegal abortion than die in the whole of the UK from legal abortion in 1 year.

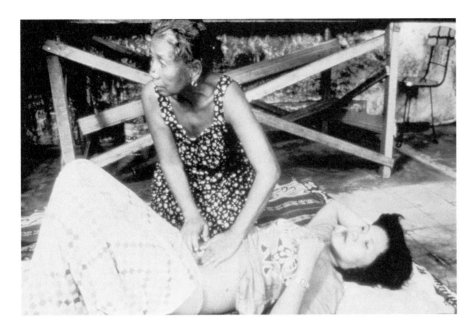

Figure 13.6 A massage abortion in the Philippines. (Photo: Joe Cantrell)

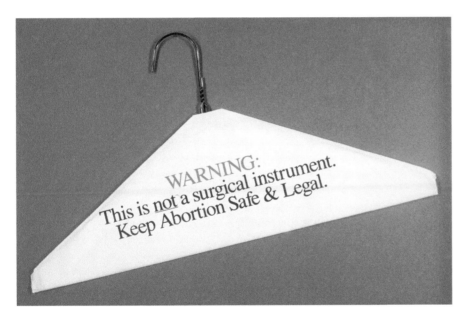

WARNING:
This is <u>not</u> a surgical instrument.
Keep Abortion Safe & Legal.

Figure 13.7 Wire from a coat hanger, which, in some countries of the developing world where abortion is illegal, is inserted into the uterus to terminate pregnancy.

All societies have a variety of abortion techniques, from the use of drugs to the insertion of foreign bodies into the cervix. Techniques of unsafe abortion include pushing foreign bodies into the cervix, taking dangerous poisons such as ergot or high doses of quinine, and physical trauma to the abdomen until the placenta is dislodged and the fetus dies (Figure 13.6). In Latin America, a urinary catheter, or 'sonda', pushed through the cervix is a common method of mechanical abortion. Umbrella ribs, the proverbial coat hanger (Figure 13.7), and sticks, twigs, roots, and even condoms that are inserted into the uterus and then filled with water have all been used to terminate pregnancy in some countries of the developing world where abortion is illegal. Physical violence to the pregnant woman is cited as a cause of abortion in the Bible (Exodus 21: 22). It is the only explicit mention of induced abortion in the Bible and, importantly, abortion is not considered murder unless the woman is killed in the process.

It is important to note that most illegal abortionists do not attempt to empty the uterus but try to induce uterine bleeding, knowing that the public hospital will then care for the woman, performing a uterine curettage. MVA with the

Karman syringe is not only proving the optimum surgical method for early abortion but is also the optimum way of treating most incomplete abortions. Instead of requiring a general anesthetic and an overnight stay in hospital after curettage with metal instruments in a fully equipped operating theater, most incomplete abortions can be treated with MVA without an anesthetic and without an overnight stay, reducing the risks to the woman and the costs to the hospital.

A MIDDLE GROUND

After a great deal of debate, the 1994 Cairo International Conference on Population and Development addressed the issue of unsafe abortion as a public health problem, stating:

> In no case should abortion be promoted as a method of family planning. All Governments and relevant intergovernmental and non-governmental organizations are urged to strengthen their commitment to women's health, to deal with the health impact of unsafe abortion as a major public health concern and to reduce the recourse to abortion through expanded and improved family planning services. Prevention of unwanted pregnancies must always be given the highest priority and all attempts should be made to eliminate the need for abortion. Women who have unwanted pregnancies should have ready access to reliable information and compassionate counseling. Any measures or changes related to abortion within the health system can only be determined at the national or local level according to the national legislative process. In circumstances in which abortion is not against the law, such abortion should be safe. In all cases, women should have access to quality services for the management of complications arising from abortion. Post-abortion counseling, education and family planning services should be offered promptly which will also help to avoid repeat abortions.

REFERENCE

1. World Health Organization. Preventing Maternal Death. Geneva: WHO, 1989.

CHAPTER 14

AIDS

Acquired immunodeficiency syndrome (AIDS) was first described as a clinical entity at the beginning of the 1980s. During 2006 around 4 million adults and children became infected with HIV (human immunodeficiency virus), the virus that causes AIDS. By the end of the year, an estimated 39.5 million people worldwide were living with HIV/AIDS. The year also saw around 3 million deaths from AIDS, despite recent improvements in access to antiretroviral treatment. Today, it is estimated that around 40 million people are infected with HIV, about the same number of people as were killed as combatants and civilians in the Second World War. Every country now has an epidemic in high risk groups of men who have sex with men (MSM), commercial sex workers (CSW) and intravenous drug users. In parts of sub-Saharan Africa there are generalized hetero-sexual epidemics (Table 14.1).

The human toll of AIDS is staggering:

- At the end of 2005, UNAIDS estimates that nearly 40 million men, women, and children worldwide were living with HIV/AIDS.

- Since the beginning of the pandemic 25 years ago, more than 25 million people have died of AIDS. Although there are antiretroviral medications now available to treat HIV infection, these drugs are not cures, and they remain out of the reach of most people who could benefit from them.
- Young people account for half of all new HIV infections worldwide – around 6000 become infected with HIV every day.[1]
- In 2005, over 4 million people became infected with HIV.

In certain severely affected countries, deaths from AIDS are seriously reducing the expectation of life: in Zambia, for example, a child has less chance of surviving past the age of 30 years today than a child born in England in 1840! Despite advances in the development of antiretroviral agents that are highly effective in containing the disease, AIDS still remains an incurable and apparently universally lethal disease. A great deal of research has been carried out in the search for a suitable vaccine, but none is yet in sight. Figure 14.1 illustrates the sequence of the formation of an

Table 14.1 Regional statistics for HIV and AIDS, end of 2006

Region	Adults and children living with HIV/AIDS	Adults and children newly infected	Adult prevalence[a]	Deaths of adults and children
Sub-Saharan Africa	24.7 million	2.8 million	5.9%	2.1 million
North Africa and Middle East	460 000	68 000	0.2%	36 000
South and South-East Asia	7.8 million	860 000	0.6%	590 000
East Asia	750 000	100 000	0.1%	43 000
Oceania	81 000	7 100	0.4%	4 000
Latin America	1.7 million	140 000	0.5%	65 000
Caribbean	250 000	27 000	1.2%	19 000
Eastern Europe and Central Asia	1.7 million	270 000	0.9%	84 000
Western and Central Europe	740 000	22 000	0.3%	12 000
North America	1.4 million	43 000	0.8%	18 000
Global total	39.5 million	4.3 million	1.0%	2.9 million

[a] Proportion of adults aged 15–49 years old who were living with HIV/AIDS.

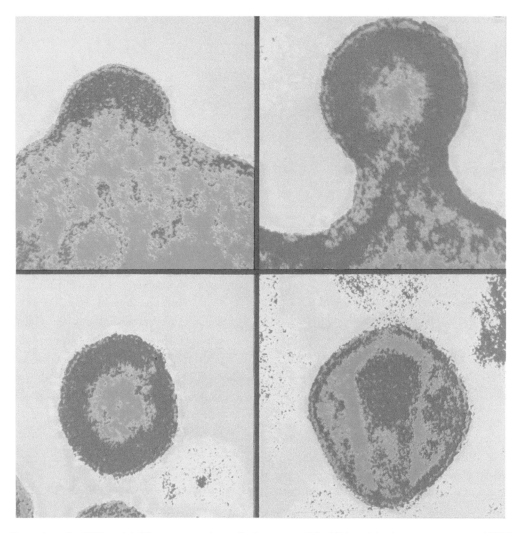

Figure 14.1 Formation of an HIV particle. The sequence shows the formation of the HIV particle, the causative agent of AIDS, on the surface of an infected lymphocyte. (Courtesy of Science Photo Library, London, UK.)

HIV particle, the causative agent of AIDS, at the surface of an infected lymphocyte.

AIDS is a disease of paradoxes. The virus itself is extremely fragile, yet it is the most lethal virus known to medicine, killing 98% or more of those it infects. HIV is relatively difficult to transmit from person to person and it can only survive in blood, semen, vaginal secretions, or milk. HIV infection never killed anyone. Death occurs as a result of opportunistic infections that occur as natural immunity crumbles owing to the HIV infection that selectively attacks T cells in the lymphoid system. The good news about HIV is that it is not transmitted by coughing and sneezing like its cousin the common cold retrovirus. Modes of transmission of HIV include blood transfusion, contaminated needles, mother-to-fetus transmission, and anal, vaginal, and oral intercourse. The most common mode of transmission is sexual.

Table 14.2 shows the global importance of each major route of HIV infection.[2]

Blood-borne transmission, particularly from needle sharing by intravenous drug users, is an exceptionally high-risk activity, and drug users often represent one of the first core groups to become infected as the disease spreads (as occurred in Thailand in the late 1980s). Anal intercourse is more likely to transmit the virus than vaginal, and vaginal intercourse is more likely to transmit the virus than oral. Men who have sex with men, and commercial sex workers, along with intravenous drug users, form the 'core groups' where the infection spreads first. The presence of certain sexually transmissible diseases, particularly those causing genital ulceration such as herpes, substantially encourages HIV transmission during sexual intercourse.

It has been known for over a decade that groups such as Moslems or Catholics in the Philippines, where the men are

Table 14.2 Mode of transmission and proportion of cumulative adult HIV infections

Type of exposure	Percent of global total
Blood transfusion	3–5
Perinatal	5–10
Sexual intercourse:	70–80
Vaginal	60–70
Anal	5–10
Injecting drug use (sharing needles, etc.)	5–10
Health care (needlestick injury, etc.)	<0.01

From reference 2.

Table 14.3 An 'anatomical vaccine': male circumcision slows the acquisition of HIV infection

	Exposure (months)			
	0–3	4–12	13–21	Total
Circumcised	2	7	11	20
Uncircumcised	9	15	25	49

From reference 3.

circumcised, have a lower rate of heterosexual HIV/AIDS than populations where men are uncircumcised. A well-designed study in South Africa in 2005 (where some men were randomly assigned to circumcision on entering the study and others 18 months later) produced such a statistically compelling result that it was felt unethical to continue the study.[3]

The inside of the foreskin is poorly keratinized and HIV attaches preferentially to the numerous Langerhans' cells embedded in the epithelium. Male circumcision has been called 'an anatomical vaccine' (Table 14.3) because unlike behavior change or the use of condoms, which have to be continually reinforced, the foreskin does not jump back on during moments of sexual passion and the protective effect (a 50% reduction in the chance of infection) is present at every intercourse.

Diseases, like people, have a reproductive rate (Figure 14.2): i.e. the number of people one person with the disease will infect before they die or recover. If the reproductive rate is above one, the disease spreads; if it is below one, it will fade out. In Africa and parts of Asia the reproductive rate for HIV infection is above one and spread is rapid. Among many heterosexual communities in the West it may be below one, which means that clusters of infection will occur by spread from groups with high-risk behaviors (e.g. intravenous drug users), although a self-sustaining epidemic is less likely. This means that even relatively small changes in behavior, condom use, or sexually transmissible disease control could have a marked effect on the overall epidemic (Figure 14.3).

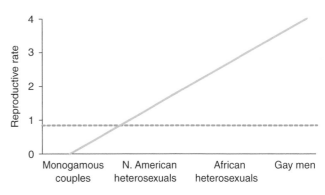

Figure 14.2 Reproductive rate of HIV.

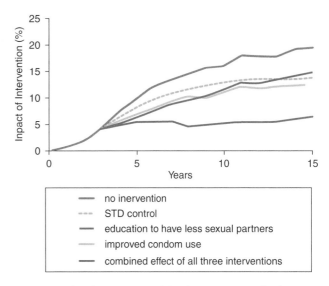

Figure 14.3 Computer model of the impact of education, improved condom use, and sexually transmissible disease (STD) control on the spread of AIDS; individually, each intervention has little impact, but all three factors together have a powerful effect.

There are four things that can be done to slow the spread of HIV:

1. Educate about the nature of the disease and the need to avoid multiple sex partners; especially concurrent sexual partners.
2. Ensure easy availability of condoms.
3. Treat other sexually transmissible diseases.
4. Offer circumcision and information about HIV transmission to those men who wish to have the operation.

Studies have shown that most people have relatively few sexual partners in a lifetime (Figure 14.4); however, a few have large numbers.

These four interventions act synergistically. There is a tremendous advantage in creating interventions as early as possible in the history of the epidemic (Figure 14.5) and

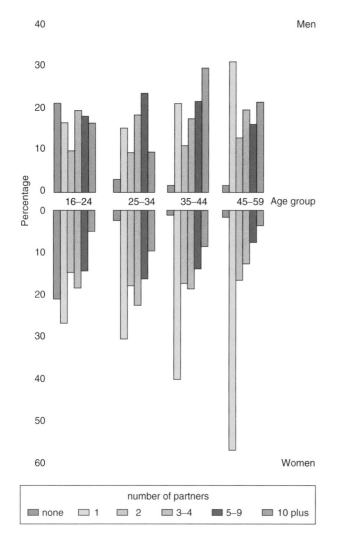

Figure 14.4   AIDS spreads partly because human sexual behavior is heterogeneous. (From reference 4.)

focusing on those individuals at highest risk of acquiring and transmitting the disease, namely sex workers and men who have sex with men.

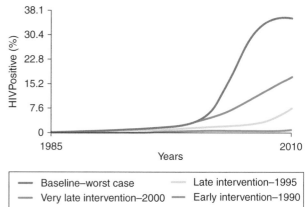

Figure 14.5   Computer model of the impact of interventions by the time the interventions are started after the beginning of an epidemic in a country. (From reference 5, with permission.)

The Millennium Development Goals, which were established by the Millennium Declaration at the United Nations in 2000, formulated a target to 'have halted by 2015 and begun to reverse the spread of HIV/AIDS'.[6] In some countries with generalized epidemics, such as Uganda, the prevalence of the disease has begun to fall. Part of this is due to welcome changes in behavior, but part is characteristic of any epidemic, where numbers rise as a large number of susceptible people are infected and then fall as they die. In the case of an infectious disease such as influenza, an epidemic can sweep through a community in a number of months. In the case of AIDS the average time between infection and death is 8 to 10 years, so it has taken a long time for the epidemic to peak.

AIDS AND FAMILY PLANNING

AIDS is changing the face of family planning, and experience from family planning is contributing to HIV/AIDS prevention. AIDS prevention uses condoms and the same range of political and counseling skills that has been used in

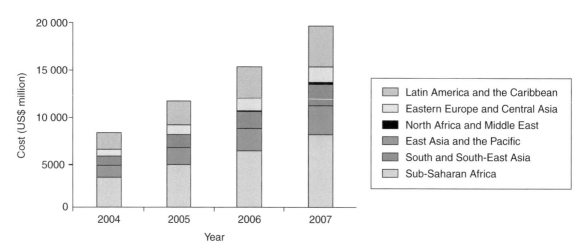

Figure 14.6   Estimated annual Projected HIV and AIDS financing needs by region, 2004–2007. (From reference 7, with permission.)

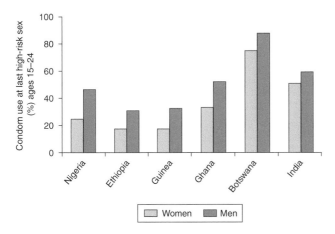

Figure 14.7 'Condom use at last high-risk sex' among 15–24 year olds in various countries (1998–2003). (From reference 8.)

the development of family planning services. Like many aspects of family planning, such as safe abortion or access to contraception for adolescents, AIDS has created a great deal of controversy, fear, and discrimination against people with the virus. It has also produced inspiring examples of leadership, compassion, and community support.

As occurred in family planning, governments have been slow to recognize the scale of the need to help poor and vulnerable groups and, globally, too little money is being spent on preventing the spread of AIDS. The estimated global cost of AIDS prevention and care for 2004 was around US$8 billion, whereas only approximately US$6 billion was actually spent in that year. For the year 2005, it was projected that a total of US$20 billion would be spent to combat HIV and AIDS (Figure 14.6).

Latex condoms significantly interrupt vaginal and anal transmission, but as HIV transmission, unlike conception, can occur on any day of the ovarian cycle, condoms must be used consistently (about 80% or more of exposed intercourses) to have a real impact on the spread of HIV. Recently, the female condom has also come into focus as an effective method of preventing HIV transmission, although cost is a deterrent to its use in poor countries. Spontaneous risky sexual acts without the use of condoms still remain a major problem amongst young people throughout the world (Figure 14.7), and the female condom can be inserted hours before sexual contact.

Vaginal spermicides such as nonoxynol-9 (N-9), which were previously believed to be effective as microbicides in combating the HIV virus, are no longer recommended for use as they may actually accelerate transmission of the virus through their irritant effects on the vaginal mucosa, which may lead to genital ulceration. N-9-impregnated condoms should not be used.

In recent years considerable investment has been made into slowing the vertical transmission of the virus from an infected mother to her newborn infant. The counseling of pregnant women and use of antiretroviral drugs during delivery is worthwhile, but needs to be supplemented by a greater emphasis on voluntary family planning. Economic analysis shows that in a society with a high prevalence of HIV, meeting the unmet need for family planning (which inevitably includes many HIV-positive mothers) is the most cost-effective way of preventing vertical transmission of HIV.

As so often happens in the analysis of anything related to human sexuality, false connections have been drawn between family planning and AIDS prevention. It has been implied

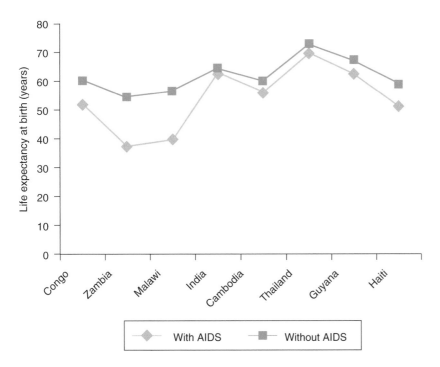

Figure 14.8 Life expectancy at birth, (both sexes combined) 2000–2005, with AIDS and without AIDS in selected countries. (From reference 9.)

that family planning is 'not needed' in some countries because so many people are going to die of AIDS. In fact, although family planning is important in reducing the birth rate, the motivation for making family planning available is to offer people the choices they want. Furthermore, even if this were not true, despite the tragic loss of life, AIDS will have little overall impact on population growth. The 40 million people likely to die from AIDS in the first decade of the current century will be equivalent to less than 6 months' population growth in that same 10 years. Finally, it must be emphasized that, unlike most infections which kill first the young and the old, HIV/AIDS kills people during their most productive years as workers and parents (Figure 14.8).

REFERENCES

1. UNAIDS/WHO AIDS Epidemic Update: December 2006. (Published in Geneva, Switzerland, UNAIDS, 2006.)
2. BMJ 2001; 322(7296): 1226–9.
3. Auvert B, Taljaard D, Lagarde E et al. Randomized, controlled intervention trial of male circumcision for reduction of HIV infection risk: the ANRS 1265 Trial. PLoS Med 2005; 2(11): e298.
4. UK Survey of Sexual Behaviour, 1992.
5. Adapted from: Influence of Mathematical Modeling of HIV and AIDS on Policies and Programs in the Developing World. Stover JMA, from The Futures Group International, Glastonbury, Connecticut USA, November 2000.
6. United Nations Millennium Declaration. Millennium Development Goals. United Nations A/RES/55/2 General Assembly September 18, 2000. Fifty-fifth session, Agenda item 60 (b) 00 55951. Resolution adopted by the General Assembly [without reference to a Main Committee (A/55/L.2)] 55/2.
7. UNAIDS. Financing the Response to AIDS 2004. http://www.unaids.org/bangkok2004/GAR2004_html/GAR2004_10_en.htm#P 1227_268579
8. UNDP. Human Development Report, 2005. http://hdr.undp.org/reports/global/2005/pdf/HDR05_complete.pdf
9. World Population Prospects. The 2004 Revision, Highlights. ESA/P/WP.193. New York: United Nations Department of Economics and Social Affairs, Population Division. February 24, 2005.

CHAPTER 15

New methods

CONTRACEPTIVE DEVELOPMENT

Contraceptive development is a long, slow, expensive, uncertain process (Figure 15.1). Thousands of chemical entities need to be screened before any are found to be effective, even in experimental animals. Of those methods which pass laboratory testing, very few are safe enough to be tested on human volunteers. In phase I clinical trials, a few tens of individuals in carefully controlled situations are given the candidate drug or device for short-term use. In phase II clinical trials a few hundred volunteers may use the method, primarily to discover any short-term hazards. In phase III clinical trials of a contraceptive, an aggregate of at least 600 woman-years of exposure is achieved and the goal is to measure effectiveness and gather additional information on short-term side effects. Once a drug has been approved for marketing, it is essential to continue postmarketing surveillance (sometimes called phase IV clinical trials). If, for example, the drug has a serious adverse effect in one in 10 000 or one in 100 000, then it may require several million woman-years of exposure before the risk is observed and measured. In today's world, it may cost US$200 million or more to bring a drug from a laboratory to the market place (Figure 15.2).

The US National Academy of Science has recently suggested that the requirements for premarketing testing of drugs might be somewhat simplified and a greater investment, including perhaps a contribution from the pharmaceutical industry, should be made in postmarketing surveillance. Postmarketing surveillance takes several years to implement, so when drugs or devices are improved, as has happened with pills and intrauterine devices (IUDs), there is often a long interval when today's methods continue to be assessed on yesterday's statistics.

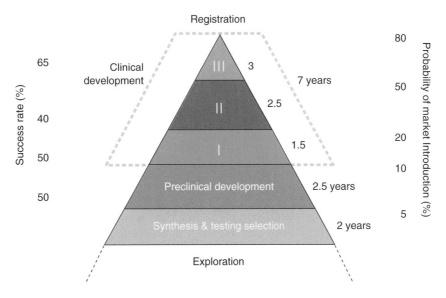

Figure 15.1 Time and risks involved in pharmaceutical research and development. (Courtesy of Professor H Vemer, NV Organon, Oss, The Netherlands.)

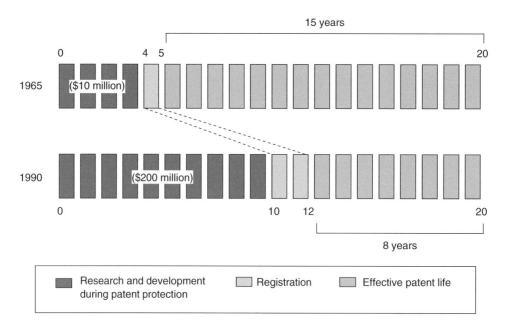

Figure 15.2 Effective patent life of medicines (1965–1990). (Courtesy of Professor H Vemer, NV Organon, Oss, The Netherlands.)

Species differences in reproduction are much wider than those for the cardiovascular system. Giving a contraceptive at several times the human dose to primates for long intervals is part of drug development but it remains an imperfect model of human physiology. In the final analysis, all new drugs and devices constitute an experiment on our own species. A great deal of patient and prudent work can be done to make the introduction of a new drug as safe as possible but there is no way to eliminate all unforeseen risks. All manipulation of the reproductive system in the prevention of unwanted pregnancy involves possible hazards and these are reflected by exceedingly high malpractice insurance rates in the USA in recent years – one reason why contraceptive pills cost $20 to over $40 dollars/cycle in the USA while the same products can be bought internationally in bulk for about 20 cents.

In the past, many companies within the pharmaceutical industry were active in genuinely innovative research and development: today, there are far fewer.

IMPROVING EXISTING METHODS

Over recent decades, improvements in existing methods have often been more important than the introduction of new methods. For example, today's IUDs and oral contraceptives are so different from the first generation of these methods introduced in the 1960s that they almost count as new methods. Incremental improvements in design are most likely when comparative studies of different methods are conducted by independent observers, as has happened

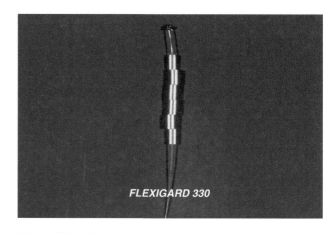

Figure 15.3 Flexigard 330, a copper-bearing IUD.

with IUDs. When first introduced, the pill used almost as much hormone in each tablet as today's user receives in a month and, as a consequence of this reduction, cardiovascular risks have been greatly reduced or even eliminated. Copper- and progestin-releasing IUDs have lower pregnancy rates and fewer side-effects than the inert plastic devices introduced 30 years ago, and the progestin-containing IUDs may actually reduce, rather than increase, the risk of pelvic inflammatory disease. The new levonorgestrel IUD also has a protective effect against the occurrence of ectopic pregnancy. New copper-bearing IUDs, for example, Flexigard 330 (Figure 15.3), may reduce the incidence of side effects.

METHODS UNDER DEVELOPMENT

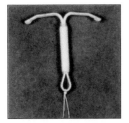

Levonorgestrel-IUD

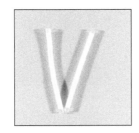

NORPLANT-2

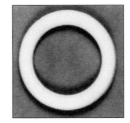

Contraceptive rings

Figure 15.4 Examples of other contraceptive methods that have been developed. (Source: Population Council, New York, USA.)

Oral contraceptive doses are unlikely to be lowered further, although new synthetic hormones may be synthesized. New implants and injectables are possible: subdermal implants with one rod instead of six would be a step forward and a biodegradable implant that did not require removal would be welcome. Steroid hormones are rapidly absorbed through the vaginal wall and even the ordinary pill has been used this way. This method of delivery bypasses the liver and has some advantages over oral use, reducing, for example, complaints of nausea. Silastic vaginal rings containing hormones have been used as successful contraceptives in WHO-sponsored trials. The levonorgestrel IUD, the subdermal implant Norplant-2, and a contraceptive ring are illustrated in Figure 15.4. Unfortunately, even simple improvements are sometimes too costly to introduce past modern drug regulatory authorities: for example, the addition of small quantities of testosterone to an injectable progestin would correct the risk of osteoporosis and reduced libido associated with the method.

IUDs, such as the device by Wildermeersch in Belgium which anchors a thread with copper sleeves in the uterus but does away with a rigid framework, may represent an important advance. Even new condoms, such as loose-fitting plastic devices, could improve the range of contraceptive choices.

DEVELOPING NEW METHODS

Theoretically, it should be possible to make a contraceptive vaccine, although unlike antibodies against an infective organism, the protein identified as the target for the vaccine must have no other natural function. The zona pellucida surrounding the egg is a unique antigen as are the gonadotropic hormones produced in the placenta which differ in their molecular structure from the corresponding hormones manufactured in the pituitary. However, the complexity of the topic and lack of funds has stalled research.

In the 1960s, when condoms and coitus interruptus were the most common methods, family planning leaders were pleading for research on female methods. Today, the cry is often to introduce a 'male pill'. WHO trials of a male systemic method using testosterone have been conducted. Testosterone is made in the Leydig cells in the testis and sperm production occurs only in an environment exposed to high levels of testosterone. If testosterone is given by injection, the pituitary gonadotropins are inhibited and, while the levels of circulating testosterone are adequate for all the other aspects of male behavior, levels in the testis fall so low that sperm production stops. It takes 120 days to make a sperm, so male systemic methods take some time to act and some time to reverse. In the case of the woman, systemically active methods imitate the natural process of ovulation inhibition occurring with pregnancy and lactation, but in the case of the man there is no natural interruption of fertility to imitate. Therefore, there are no biological reasons for assuming a male systemic method might have any advantages of the sort associated with the pill and reduction of cancer. High doses of testosterone, however, can cause aggressive behavior in men. A variety of chemicals have been tried that prevent sperm production or interfere with specific components of sperm activity, such as acrosome function, but development has been suspended because of costs and uncertain outcomes.

Hypothalamic releasing hormones have been well studied in women and men and are relatively easy to synthesize. At first glance, they offer little advantage over pituitary hormones, other than interrupting the same reproductive processes at a different location. However, Pike and his co-workers in Los Angeles are exploring a combination of hypothalamic releasing and ovarian hormones, designed not only to inhibit fertility but also to change the hormonal environment of the breast in such a way as to reduce the risk of cancer later in life. It will require time and large-scale use to demonstrate if either of these approaches reduces breast cancer, but if either succeeds, it is likely to form the basis of a new generation of fundamentally different and profoundly important therapies for the 21st century.

Unfortunately, the monies going into new methods are insufficient to bring about any real revolution in family planning in the near future. Probably the best that can be hoped for is a slow but steady improvement in current methods and perhaps some new barrier methods to fill the need mentioned earlier for a method women could use to protect themselves against HIV and other sexually transmissible diseases.

CHAPTER 16

Conclusions

Those who believe reproductive freedom is a basic human right are beginning to emerge from a long dark tunnel: for the first time in human history, there are one or two regions of the world where women enjoy social equality with men, sexual autonomy, and freedom of reproductive choice. In other, larger areas of the world change is occurring and progress is being made, but elsewhere hundreds of millions of women remain disadvantaged, often exploited and sometimes emotionally or physically abused. Where women are unjustly treated, men cannot reach their full potential either.

It may take generations before the bonds of tradition are broken in some places. Fortunately, family planning choices can be made available relatively quickly and in almost any culture, from the Islamic areas of South Asia, where many women are in purdah, to the single mother with a series of partners, encountered in the Caribbean. While access to family planning cannot solve social or economic problems, it can lighten the heavy burdens laid on people – especially women – by their circumstances. Indeed, surveys have shown that millions of women do not want more children (Figure 16.1).

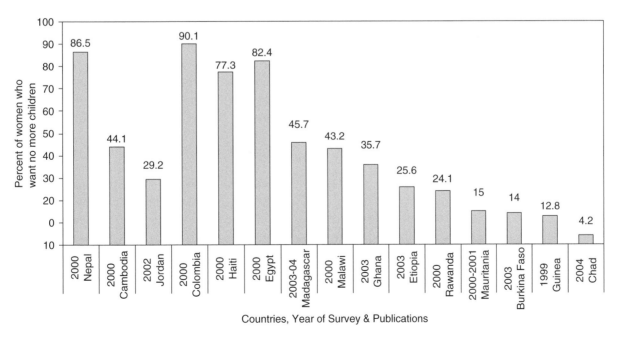

Figure 16.1   Desire to stop childbearing among currently married women with three living children. (From reference 1.)

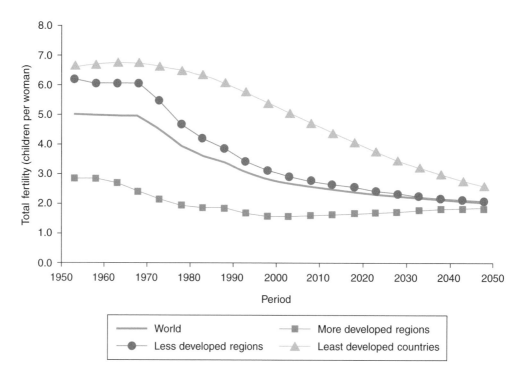

Figure 16.2 Total fertility trajectories of the world and major development groups, 1950–2050 (medium variant). (From reference 3.)

Around the world, over 600 million married women are using contraception – nearly 500 million in developing countries. Fertility fell in almost all developing countries surveyed since 1990, as use of modern contraception rose. These trends continue a long-term change in attitudes and behavior. Findings from more than 100 surveys conducted since 1990 suggest that, as family planning programs have become widespread, more and more people want smaller families, and more succeed in having the size of family that they want.[2]

Many countries have shown a rapid decline in fertility reduction. Those countries having the fastest fertility reductions between 1970–1975 and 2000–2005 are mostly in Asia, Iran (66.8%), Kuwait (65.5%), Mongolia (66.6%), Thailand (61.2%), the Republic of Korea (71.4%), and Vietnam (65.3%), but they also include Algeria (65.7%) and Tunisia (67.8%) in Northern Africa and Mexico (63.6%) in Latin America (Figure 16.2).

The pace and extent to which family planning choices are expanded not only have a profound impact on the reproductive health of individuals but also have an important relationship with other global problems, particularly related to the environment and to the huge task of moving the global economy from its present dependence on fossil fuels to one that is biologically sustainable.

The difficulty of recreating the cloying conservatism that held back family planning in the Western world until the second half of the 20th century has been emphasized earlier. In the 1920s, Aldous Huxley said of his contemporary world, 'In most countries, the only state-supported orthodoxy is sexual orthodoxy'. Only the strongest and most charismatic of personalities were able to break through the formidable barriers which society had built between individuals and their reproductive freedoms. Those who fought for family planning were not always likeable people: Marie Stopes was a prima donna who frequently quarreled with her colleagues; Helena Wright had an eccentric belief in spiritualism; and Margaret Sanger, like all of us, was a prisoner of her own time. She wrote about 'illiterates, paupers, unemployables, criminals, prostitutes, dope-fiends' whom she felt should be separated from the rest of society to 'improve their moral conduct' and prevent them reproducing.

Until the 1970s demographers had little accurate information on contraceptive usage and even today some continue to ignore the role of abortion in fertility decline because data on this important variable are necessarily weak. In the classic theory of the demographic transition, differentials in fertility between different social groups or different countries were explained by differences in education, income, and other variables where solid data were available. It followed that, if these differentials could not be removed, there would have to be some degree of coercion. As late as 1952, at the time of the foundation of the International Planned Parenthood Federation, a distinguished scientist, Professor Joseph Needham, believed only compulsion would lower fertility in some countries.

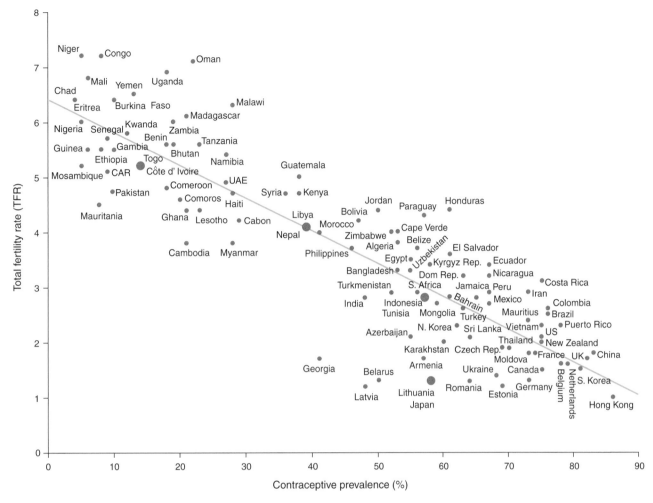

Figure 16.3 The relationship between fertility and contraceptive use. 105 countries surveyed between 1990–2001. TFR: the average number of children a woman would have during her lifetime if current age-specific fertility rates remained constant over her reproductive years. Contraceptive prevalence: the percentage of married women ages 15–49 using any method of contraception (not including folk or traditional methods other than withdrawal and periodic abstinence).

The glorious discovery of the past 40 years has been that, when individuals of any social, ethnic, or cultural background are given genuine choices, then the overwhelming majority does not choose to have more children than their love and physical resources can support.

Family planning needs promotion, just as the soft-drink industry or soap powders need promotion, but to succeed it should be targeted at individual perceptions and personal needs. The 'unemployables', whose large families worried Margaret Sanger, were simply those who had even less opportunity than their neighbors of jumping over the many hurdles separating them from the family planning services that they needed. The rapid growth of developing countries that worried Joseph Needham was, to a considerable extent, a manifestation of the fact that Europeans denied their colonies access to family planning, even more thoroughly than they tried to deny it to their own citizens.

The light at the end of the tunnel is growing brighter but is still some way off. Contemporary family planning policies are often muddled. Some decision-makers still repeat yesterday's mistakes and assume that fertility will not decline until other variables, such as education and income, are improved. Obviously, family planning moves more rapidly in a world where people are literate and prosperous, but socioeconomic progress is not a prerequisite of a falling birth rate. Even in the West, research shows that the advent of the pill has had more effect on fertility decline than economic change.

When international family planning began in the 1960s, rapid population growth was recognized as a problem, but no one really knew what would be the 'solution'. Some experts wrote of 'beyond family planning', and 'incentives' were discussed. Today, even though some people still fight over yesterday's shadows, there has been a wonderful coming

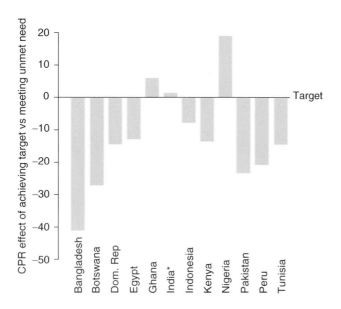

Figure 16.4 Contraceptive prevalence rate (CPR) effect of achieving target vs meeting unmet need. (From reference 4, with permission.)

together of those who support family planning as an individual choice and as an effective health intervention.

Voluntary family planning programs also had a profound effect on explosive population growth. Meeting all the unmet need for family planning could bring the final stable population of the planet to one-half of the level it would have been without 30 years of international effort (Figure 16.3). The people have voted for reproductive freedom with pills, condoms, intrauterine devices, and sterilization. People all over the world have demonstrated that they want modern family planning. Indeed, the unmet need for family planning usually exceeds the demographic 'targets' set by governments. In Bangladesh, people, of their own volition, want 40% fewer children than the most ambitious targets demographers had conceived for the country. Figure 16.4 compares the demographic targets with the unmet need in 12 countries; a negative number indicates that the satisfaction of unmet need would result in a contraceptive prevalence rate higher than that set by policymakers based on purely demographic considerations.

Most sensible people accept that another doubling of the global population is going to put many strains on the world that our children inherit, but the 'solution' is not to try to persuade people to make decisions for the common good, but to make choices in their own self-interest and for love of their family.

REFERENCES

1. Demographic and Health Surveys. Studies in family planning.
2. Population Reports Volume XXXI, Number 2, Spring 2003. Series M, Number 17, Special Topics.
3. Population Division of the Department of Economic and Social Affairs of the United Nations Secretariat (2005). World Population Prospects: The 2004 Revision. Highlights. New York: United Nations.
4. Senanayake P, Kleinman RL. Family Planning Meeting Challenges, Promoting Choices. Carnforth, UK: Parthenon, 1992.

Index

Note: Page references in *italic* refer to illustrations or tables

abortion, induced 15, 31
  and contraceptive use 95, *97*
  ethical issues 95, 97
  laws 95, *96*
  mortality *97, 98*
  opinions 95
  rape victims 93
  and religious beliefs 15, *16*
  safe techniques 97–8
  unsafe 98–100, *99*
  worldwide incidence *97*
  in young women 84
abortion, spontaneous 6, *7*
access to contraception 33–7, 113–14
  and abortion rate 95
  barriers 14, 34, *34*
  community-based services 36–7, *36, 37*
  role of health personnel 33–4
adolescents 83–6
  biological basis of behavior 83–4
  choice of contraceptives 84–6
  pregnancy rates *8*, 84, *85*
  pregnancy risks 8–9, *8, 9*
  premarital coitus *32*
  rights 84
  worldwide fertility *8*
Africa 112
  adolescent fertility *8*
  condom use *58*
  HIV/AIDS *101*, 103
  maternal deaths *13*
  unsafe abortion 98, *99*
  see also named countries and regions
age
  at first pregnancy *4*
  at first sexual intercourse *32*
  at marriage 8, *9, 32*, 84, *85*
  at puberty/menarche 2–4, *3, 4*, 84, *85*
  WHO contraception eligibility criteria *91*
AIDS/HIV 90
  'ABC' of prevention 59
  condom use 59
  costs of prevention and care *104*, 105
  deaths from 101, *101*
  and family planning 104–6

first described 101
  and life expectancy *105*, 106
  and spermicides 61, 105
  transmission 102–4
  vertical transmission 105
Albania *10*
Algeria 112
Allendale Pharmaceutical Company 62
anatomy
  female reproductive 29
  male reproductive *27, 79*
Anglican religion 21
Angola *58*
Armenia *10*
arterial disease, risk of 86, *86*, 90
Asia
  adolescent fertility *8*
  condom use *58*
  HIV/AIDS *101*, 103
  maternal deaths *13*
  tsunami disaster 90, 92, 93
  see also named countries
Augustine, Saint 21, 74

Baker, Dr JR 23
Bangladesh *58*, 78, 87, *88*, 114, *114*
barrier contraceptives, female 61
  cervical cap 62–3, *63*
  diaphragms 63–4
  female condom 64–6, *65*
  Lea's shield 64, *64*
  spermicides 61, *61*
  sponges 61–2, *62*
  use in older women 87
  use in selected countries *35*
  use in young people 86
barrier contraceptives, male, *see* condoms
Beijing Declaration and Platform for Action 84
Benin *32*
Bernadine of Sienna, Saint 75
Besant, Annie 21
Bible 21, 99
'biosocial gap' 84, *85*
birth order *11*
birth rates
  and abortion laws 95
  and contraceptive use 15

birth spacing 2, 12
  and breastfeeding 2, 29, 31, *31*, 87–8, *87*
  and child development 12, *12*
  and infant mortality *11*
  and perinatal outcome *12*
block pessary 24–5, *24*
blood pressure, raised, *see* hypertension
Bolivia *32*
bone mineral density, adolescents 85
Botswana *114*
Bradlaugh, Charles 21
brain
  development in child/adolescent 83
  and sexual behavior 27
Brazil *58*, 78
breast cancer
  death rates *43*
  risk factors 4, *4*, 29
  risk and hormonal contraception 41–2, *43*, 109–10
breastfeeding 2, 29–31
  benefits of 29
  and birth spacing 2, 29, 31, *31*, 87–8, *87*
  contraception during 88–9
  return of menstruation/ovulation 87–8, *87*
Bulgaria *10*

Cairo International Conference on Population and Development 84, 100
calendar (rhythm) method 71, *72*, 74
Cambodia *10*, *111*
cancer risks 4, *4*, 29, *81*
  female sterilization 81, *81*
  oral contraceptive use 41–4, *43*, 109–10
carbon dioxide emissions *17*
cardiac disease 90
cardiovascular risk, oral contraceptives 86, *86*
Caribbean *8*, *13*, *58*, *101*, 111
Casanova 24
Catholic religion 15, *16*, 21, 23, 74
Ceauşescu, Nicolae 95
cervical cancer risk 42–3
cervical cap 62–3, *63*
cervical mucus
  effects of oral contraceptives 44–5, 47
  ovulation detection 71, 73–4, *73*
cervix 29
  self-palpation 74
cesarean section 78
Chad *111*
Chang, MC 39
childbearing
  desire to stop 18–19, *19*, *111*
  women's health risk 2, 4
children
  development and birth spacing 12, *12*, *13*
  health and high-risk pregnancies 9, 14
  number, *see* birth spacing; family size
Chile *97*
chimpanzees 27, 28
China *58*, 70, 78
Chlamydia trachomatis 59
Christian religions 15, *16*, 21, 23, 74
chromosomal abnormalities *7*
circumcision 102–3
clinical trials
  contraceptive development 107, *107*
  oral contraceptives 39
clinics, reproductive health 85
coitus, premarital *32*

coitus interruptus 75–6, *75*
  mentioned in bible 21
  pregnancy rates 74, *74*
  use in selected countries *35*
Collaborative Group on Hormonal
    Factors in Breast Cancer 42
Colombia *11*, *32*, *111*
Comstock, Anthony 21
Comstock laws 22
conception 6, *6*
condoms
  animal membranes 59
  education in use 57–8
  efficacy of use 58–9, *59*
  ensuring correct use of 59, *59*
  female 64–6, *65*
  manufacture 57, *57*
  origin of term 57
  plastic 58
  rubber (latex) 57
  and sexually-transmitted diseases 59, 105, *105*
  supply sources *34*
conflict, family planning introduction 22–4
consumption 17, *17*
Convention on the Elimination of all Forms of
    Discrimination against Women 84
Convention on the Rights of the Child 84
Costa Rica *11*, *58*
Counseling
  abortion 100
  female sterilization 89
  young people 85
CycleBeads 74–5, *75*

Dalkon Shield 69–70
decision-making
  in adolescents 83
  female sterilization 89
demographic transition 15–16, 112
Denmark *3*
Depo-Provera 49–50
depot medroxyprogesterone acetate (DMPA) 49, *50*, 85
developed countries
  adolescent fertility *8*
  condom use *58*
  fertility trends 112, *112*
developing countries
  access to contraception 33, *33*, *34*, 36–7, *36*, *37*
  adolescent fertility *8*
  condom use *58*, 59, *59*
  injectable contraceptives 49
  need/desire for contraception 18–19, *19*, *111*, 114, *114*
development, economic 14–15, *15*
development of contraceptives 39, 107–8, *107*
diabetes mellitus 90, *91*
diaphragms 63–4
dihydroxyprogesterone (algestone) acetophenide *50*
disabled persons 89–90
disasters, natural 90, 92–3
Dominican republic *10*
Down syndrome 9

East Asia
  adolescent fertility *8*
  HIV/AIDS statistics *101*
Eastern Europe, HIV/AIDS statistics *101*
Ebers papyrus 24, 25, 61
Ecuador *11*

education
    condom use 58
    HIV/AIDS transmission 103, *103*
Egypt *10, 58, 111, 114*
electrocautery, female sterilization 79
El Salvador *58*
embryo, abnormalities 6, *7*
emergency contraception
    humanitarian crises 92
    IUDs 70
    oral hormones 47–8, *48*
    young people 86
endometrial (uterine) cancer risk 41, 52
endometrium, effects of oral contraceptives 45, *45*
environmental change 17
equality, sexual 14, 111
Eritrea *19*
Eskimos *3*
estradiol cypionate *50*
estradiol enanthate *50*
estradiol valerate 49, *50*
estrogen
    endogenous *45*, 71
    oral contraceptives 44
ethical issues
    abortion 95, 97
    sterilization 77–8
ethinylestradiol 44
    vascular disease risk 86, *86*
Ethiopia *32*, 98, *111*
etonogestrel, implant *53*, 54
Europe, HIV/AIDS statistics *101*
evolution 28

F-5 gel 62
failure (pregnancy) rates
    cervical cap use 63
    coitus interruptus 75
    condoms 58–9
    diaphragms 64
    IUDs 69–70
    Lea's shield 64
    natural methods of contraception 74, *74*
    oral contraceptives 39
    periodic abstinence 71
Fallopian tubes, ligation/occlusion 78–9, *80*, 81
Fallopius, Gabriel 57
Family Health International 58
Family Limitation (Sanger) 22
family size
    and desire to stop childbearing 18–19, *19, 111*
    and population growth 18–19, *18*
    and risks in pregnancy 10–12, *11*
FC2 female condom 65–6
female condoms 64–6, *65*
    reuse of 66
Femcap 63
fertility
    and breastfeeding 29, 31, 87–8, *87*, 88, *88*
    and contraceptive use *113*
    possible points of intervention *1*
    trends in 112, *112*
fertility tracking
    cervical mucus method 71, 73–4, *73*
    CycleBeads 74–5
    'symptothermal' method 73
fertilization 6, *6*
Filshie clip 79, *81*

Finland *10*
Flexigard 330 IUD 108, *108*
Florey, Professor Howard 23
follicle stimulating hormone (FSH) 28, 44–5, *44, 45*
Food and Drug Administration (FDA) 23
foreskin, HIV transmission 103
France *35, 58*
The Fruits of Philosophy 21

Gabon *32*
Ghana *11, 19, 32, 111, 114*
Guinea *111*

Haberlandt, Ludwig 39
Haiti *32*
health personnel, role in family planning 1–2, 33
heart attack 40
herpes simplex 59
history of family planning 21–5
HIV 102, *102*
    interventions to slow spread 103–4
    modes of transmission 102–3, *103*
    reproductive rate *103*
    see also AIDS/HIV
hormonal contraceptives
    implants 52–4
    injectables 48–52, 86, 109
    patch 54, *55*
    vaginal contraceptive ring 54–6
    see also oral contraceptives
hormonal cycles (female) 28, *29*
    alteration by contraceptives 44–6, *44, 45*
    alteration by injectable contraceptives *49*
hormone replacement therapy (HRT) 70
hormones
    adolescent 83
    lactation 29, *30*
    male 28, 109
Humanae Vitae 21
humanitarian crises 90, 92–3
human papillomavirus (HPV) 43
human rights
    children/adolescents 84
    rationale for contraception 14, 111
hunter-gatherer societies 2
Hutterites 31
Huxley, Aldous 112
17α-hydroxyprogesterone caproate *50*
hypertension 40, 90, *92*
    WHO eligibility criteria *91*
hypothalamic releasing hormones 109–10
hysterectomy, disabled woman 89

Implanon *53*, 54, *54*
implants 52–4
    advantages 52
    development 109
    drawbacks 52
    'patch' 54, *55*
    removal 54
    young people 85
India *10*, 78, *114*
Indonesia *11, 19, 114*
    2004 tsunami 90
infant mortality 2
    and birth order *11*
    and birth spacing *11*
    and maternal age *10*

injectable contraceptives 48–52
  advantages of use *52*
  development 109
  formulations, injection schedules and availability *50*
  safety studies 51–2
  use in older women 86
  young people 85
International Agency for Research on Cancer (IARC) 43
International Conference on Population and Development (ICPD) 84, 100
intrauterine devices (IUDs)
  complications of use 68–9
  contraindications 68
  copper-bearing 70, 92, *108*
  development of 67–8
  emergency contraception 70
  failure rates 69–70
  hormone-releasing 68, 70, 108–9, *109*
  in humanitarian crises 92
  improvements 108–9, *109*
  insertion 69, *69*
  mortality from 68, *68*
  in older women 86
  origins 25
  types *68*, 69
  wishbone 26, *67*
  worldwide use *35*, 70
Iran 23–4, *23*, 33, *33*, 58
Irish Family Planning Association 23
Islam 23–4, 111
Israel *10*
Italy *35*, 58

Jadelle 52–3, *53*
Japan 33, *35*, 39, *58*
Jordan *10*, *111*

Kalahari, !Khun society 2
Karman cannula *98*
Karman, Harvey 98
Kenya *10, 11, 19, 32, 58, 114*
!Khun 2
Knowlton, Charles 21
Korea, Republic of 112
Kuwait 112

lactation 29–31
lactational amenorrhea method (LAM) 29, 31, 87–9, *88, 89*
  advantages and disadvantages of 88–9, *89*
  conditions for *31*
Lambeth Conference (1920) 21
Langerhans' cells 103
Latin America
  abortion 98
  adolescent fertility *8*
  condom use *58*
  fertility trends 112
  HIV/AIDS *101*
  maternal deaths *13*
  sterilization 82
  see also named countries
Laufe, Leonard 68
Lea's shield 64, *64*
least-developed countries
  adolescent fertility *8*
  fertility trends *112*
legal issues, sterilization 77–8
levonorgestrel
  IUD 68, 70, 108–9, *109*

oral contraceptives 46, 49
  vascular disease risk 86, *86*
Levo-Nova 70
life, start of 95, 97
life expectancy
  and AIDS 101, *105*, 106
  and oral contraceptive use 43–4
liver cancer 43
lung cancer, death rates *43*
luteinizing hormone (LH) 28, 44–5, *44, 45*
lymphocyte, HIV particle formation *102*

McCormack, Paige 39
Madagascar *111*
magnetic resonance imaging
  (MRI), brain development 83
Malawi *111*
'male pill' 109
male reproductive organs *27, 79*
Mali *10, 11, 32*
manual vacuum aspiration (MVA) 98, 99–100
marriage, age at 8, *9, 32*, 84, *85*
maternal mortality 12–14, *13, 14*
  and abortion rates 95, *97*
  adolescent mothers 8, *9*
  induced abortion *97, 98*
  and parity/family size 10, *10*
  statistics *13*
mating systems 28
Mauritania *10*
medical illness, contraception during 90, *91, 92*
medroxyprogesterone acetate (MPA) 48–9
  depot 49, *50*, 85
menarche, age at 2–4, *3, 4*, 84, *85*
menopause 70, 86
  age at *4*
menorrhagia 70
menstrual cycle
  effects of implantable contraceptives 52
  effects of oral contraceptives 44–6, *45*
  predicting fertility/safe period 71–4, *71, 72, 73*
  return during breastfeeding 87–8, *87*
mestranol 44
Mexico *11*, 112
mifepristone (RU-486) 98
Millennium Development Goals (MDGs) 84
  adolescents 84
  HIV/AIDS 104
minilaparotomy 79, 81
Minimal Initial Service Package (MISP) 92
Mirena 68, 70
misoprostol 98
Mongolia 112
monogamous mating systems 28
mortality, *see* infant mortality;
    maternal mortality

Needham, Professor Joseph 112
Neisseria gonorrhoeae 59
Nepal *10, 11, 111*
Nestorone 53, *53*
NET-EN 49, *50*
Netherlands *35*, 39, 95
Nicaragua *32*
Nigeria, condom use *58*
nomegestrol acetate 53, *53*
nonoxynol-9 (N-9) 61, 62
  and HIV 105

norethindrone 47, 49, 50, *50*
Norplant-2 109, *109*
Norplant 52, *53*
North America
    HIV/AIDS statistics *101*
    see also USA
Norway *10*
NuvaRing 54–6, *55*

obesity 90
Oceania
    HIV/AIDS *101*
    maternal deaths *13*
older women
    contraception 86–7
    pregnancy/childbirth 9, *10*
    smokers 44
oral contraceptives
    access to 33, *33*
    breastfeeding 89
    cancer risk 41–3, 109–10
    combined 41, 44, *48*, 85, 86
    continuous-use 46–7, *47*
    contraindications *46*
    costs of 108
    development 39, 109
    emergency (postcoital) 47–8
    failure rates 39
    formulations, choice 40, *40*
    formulations, comparison *48*
    global use 39
    low-estrogen 44
    'male' pill 109
    missed/delayed 46, *46*, *47*
    mode of action 44–5, *44*, *45*
    non-contraceptive benefits 40–1, *41*
    progestogen-only 47, *48*, 86
    short-term advantages 45–6, *45*
    short-term disadvantages *46*
    side effects 39–41, *41*
    use in humanitarian crises 92
    world wide use *35*, 43–4
    young women 85
ova (eggs)
    fertilization *6*
    lifetime number in ovary 6, *6*
ovarian cancer risk 41, 52, 81, *81*
ovaries, lifetime number of germ cells 6, *6*
over-the-counter contraceptives
    oral 44
    sponges 62
Oves cervical cap 63
ovulation
    concealment in humans 28
    prediction of 71–4, *71*, *72*, *73*
    return in lactation 87–8, *87*
oxytocin *30*

Pakistan *11*, 14, *114*
Panama *11*
Paraguay *58*
parity, and maternal mortality 10, *10*
patch contraceptive 54, *55*
patent life, medicines *108*
pelvic inflammatory disease 68
periodic abstinence 71–4
    body temperature method 71, *71*
    cervical mucus method 71, 73–4, *73*

use in selected countries *35*
woman with irregular cycles *72*
young people 86
Peru *10, 11, 88, 114*
pessary
    block 24–5, *24*
    stem 67, *67*
pharmaceutical research 107–8, *107*, *108*
pharmacies, as source of contraceptives *34*
Philippines *11*, *32*, 102–3
physicians, role in family planning 33–4
Pincus, Gregory 39
placenta 29
pollution, and consumption *17*
Population Council 52, 53
population growth 2, *2*, 15–19
    and AIDS *105*, 106
    demographic transition 15–16, 112
    and family size 18–19, *18*
    impact of contraception 113–14, *113*, *114*
    potential 5, *5*
    United Nations prediction 15, *16*, 17
Portugal *10*
postcoital contraception, *see* emergency contraception
poverty 14, 17
pregnancy
    adolescent 8–9, *8*, *9*, 84, *85*
    age at first *4*
    diaphragm refitting 64
    health risks 10–11, *41*, *42*
    HIV transmission 105
    and medical disorders 90
    rates in lactational amenorrhea 88, *88*
    risks 7, *8*
    spontaneous abortions 6, *7*
    see also failure (pregnancy) rates
preliterate societies 2, 29
primates, non-human 27, 28
progesterone *45*, 71
progestins
    IUDs 108–9, *109*
    oral contraceptives 44, 46
    progestogen implants 52–3, *53*
    progestogen-only pill 47, *48*, 86
prolactin *30*, *44*
Protectaid sponge 62
Protestant religion 15, *16*
puberty, age of 2–4, *3*, *4*, 84, *85*

quinacrine tablet *81*

rape victims 48, 90, 92, 93, 95
Reality female condom 65
refugees 92
religions
    and abortion 15, *16*
    and family planning 21, 23, 74, 76
reproduction 27, *27*
    changing patterns 31–2, *31*, *32*
    endocrine control 28, *29*
    human behavior 27–8
    potential human 5–6
reproductive health clinics 85
rhythm (calendar) method 71, *72*, 74
rights, *see* human rights
ring, vaginal 54–6, *55*
Rock, John 39
Romania *10*, 95

Russia 95
Rwanda 90, *111*

Sachs, Sadie 21–2
Sanger, Margaret 21–2, *22*, 39, 112, 113
Seasonique 46–7, *47*
semen 5, 5, 28–9
Senegal *11*, 87, *88*
service delivery 33–7, 113–14
    community-based 36–7, *36*, *37*
    integration with medical care 34, 36
sexual behavior 27–8
    and AIDS transmission 103, *104*
sexual competition 27
sexual intercourse, age at first *32*
sexually transmitted diseases 5
    and condom use 59
    spermicide and 61, 105
Shungiang, Dr Li 78
SILCS device 64
Singapore *12*, *58*
smoking 40, 90
    and oral contraceptive use 43–4, 47
    WHO eligibility criteria *91*
social equality 14, 111
social marketing 36–7, *36*, *37*
socioeconomic factors 14, 15
'sonda' 99
South Africa *10*, 103
spacing of births, *see* birth spacing
sperm 28–9
    aging 9–10
    fertilization of egg 6, *6*
spermicides 61, *62*
    and HIV virus 61, 105
    insertion technique *61*
    use in young people 86
sponges 61–2, *62*
Sri Lanka 14, *19*, *88*
Standard Days 74
stem pessary 67, *67*
sterilization
    advantages and disadvantages *78*
    counseling 89
    ethical and legal issues 77–8
    female 78–9, *78*, *80*, 81
    male (vasectomy) 78, *78*, *79*, *80*
    in older women 87
    postpartum female 89
    regret 81–2
    reversal 93
    use in selected countries *35*
    in young people 86
Stopes, Marie 112
stroke 40
sub-Saharan Africa
    adolescent fertility *8*
    condom use *58*, 59
    HIV/AIDS *101*
    injectable contraceptives 49
    maternal deaths *13*
sustainability, transition to 17–18

Tamil Nadu, tsunami disaster 93
Tanzania *10*
testosterone
    endogenous 28, 109

injections 109
Thailand *11*, *36*, *37*, 112
    condom use *58*
    HIV/AIDS 102
Thomas Aquinas, Saint 21
thromboembolism risk
    in medical disease 90
    oral contraceptive use 47
Today sponge 62
trisomy *7*
tsunami (Asia 2004) 90, 92, 93
Tunisia *11*, 112, *114*
Turkey *58*, 76
Turkmenistan *10*

Uganda 104
UNAIDS 101
UNFPA 92
Uniplant 53, *53*
United Kingdom (UK)
    age at menarche *3*
    contraceptive use by type *35*
United States (USA)
    abortions 84, 95
    condom use *58*
    contraceptive use by type *35*
    fertility rates *15*, 17
    infant mortality and maternal age *10*
    sterilization 78
Ureaplasma urealyticum 59
US Agency for International
        Development (USAID) 49
US National Institutes of Health 23
US Supreme Court 97
uterine cancer risk 41, 52
uterine perforation 68–9
uterus 29
Uzbekistan 10

vaccine, contraceptive 109
vaginal contraceptive ring 54–6, 55
vaginal tenting 64
vascular disease 47, 86, *86*, 90
vas deferens, ligation 78, 79, 80
vasectomy 78, *78*, *79*, *80*
Vatican State 23
Vietnam 10, 81, 112
Viravaidya, Senator Mechai 37

weight change, and diaphragm fitting 63–4
withdrawal method, see coitus interruptus
women, social status 14, 111
Worcester Foundation, Boston 39
World Health Organization (WHO) 23
    eligibility criteria for contraception 90, *91*
    injectable contraceptives 51
    oral contraceptive guidance 40, 42, 48
    protocol for safe use of female condom 66
World Population Plan of Action 14
Wright, Helena 112

Young, James 97–8

Zambia 101
Zimbabwe *10*
Zipper, Jaime 81
zona pellucida *6*, 109